BEYONDPAIN

BEYONDPAIN

making the mind-body connection

with a foreword by oliver sacks

angela mailis-gagnon and david israelson

University of Michigan Press

Ann Arbor

Published by the University of Michigan Press, 2005
First published by VIKING CANADA, Penguin Group

Library of Congress Cataloging-in-Publication Data

Mailis-Gagnon, Angela.
    Beyond pain : making the mind-body connection / Angela Mailis-Gagnon and David
  Israelson ; with a foreword by Oliver Sacks.
      p. cm.
    Includes bibliographical references and index.
    ISBN 0-472-03082-5 (pbk. : alk. paper)
      1. Pain.   2. Mind and body.   I. Israelson, David.   II. Title.
  RB127.M334 2004
  616′.0472—dc22

                                                                    2004062143

To my patients:
Those whose pain I managed well and most importantly
all those I and my science have not been able to help.

To the best men of my life:
My late father . . . for the endless nights he spent silently
watching me study till the wee hours of the morning;
My teenage sons Nicholas and Alex . . . for teaching
me how to juggle motherhood, career and personal life;
My best friend and buddy, my husband Norm . . .
for growing with me every day of our life.
–Angela Mailis-Gagnon

To Susan, Jacob, Tessa and Jemma
–David Israelson

Contents

Acknowledgements

This book is based on the stories of hundreds of patients who triggered my curiosity and challenged me with symptoms and signs that did not fit what I was taught in medical school and were not written about in books. It is my patients who trained me on the job, and I am grateful for this. While all case histories in this book come from my archives and medical records, I have used assumed names, and certain details may have been changed to preserve anonymity and confidentiality.

Much of the scientific information in this book comes from the research of many scientists around the world. Without their work this book may have not been possible.

When it comes to my own research, I want to thank my colleagues, my pain team members and my students for their contributions and collaborations.

In the making of the book I would especially like to thank Dr. Keith Nicholson, Dr. Karen Davis and Dr. David Etlin for providing me with valuable comments on the scientific accuracy and validity of certain chapters. I want to thank Lori May, Susan Ewing, Lori Biduke-Harris, Margarita Umana, Marios Papagapiou and Ann Corman for reviewing parts of the book and for offering me ideas and constructive criticism. My gratitude also goes to those patients of mine who reviewed certain chapters and helped me express what I wanted to say in a language they could understand. I want to particularly recognize Anna Kenyon, my long-time friend and assistant, who has helped me immensely by reviewing book material, rearranging my busy clinic schedule when I was falling behind and offering me a sympathetic ear and sound advice during frustrating and anxious moments.

Many thanks to Beverley Slopen, who provided me with wise advice, and all the staff at Viking (including Diane Turbide, Nicole de Montbrun and Joe Zingrone) for their help and professionalism. In particular, I would like to recognize Lisa Berland for her editorial assistance. Her witty and intelligent queries provoked me to think and rethink parts of the book. Thank you, Lisa.

Finally, my greatest gratitude goes to my husband Norm and my sons Nicholas and Alex for their patience, encouragement and tolerance. My boys celebrated the end of the book with a big family outing (to make sure they could get acquainted again with the mother they lost for many months). As far as my husband is concerned, not only did he provide me with his talent and his drawings for the book, but he served as a careful listener, asking all the right questions for several chapters. I must also recognize his endless support and positive reinforcement, ranging from encouragement to threats like this: "If you continue falling behind your deadlines, I'll lock you up in your room with a tray of food and water until you are done!"

At the end, however, the ideas, concepts, interpretations of scientific data and personal biases are all mine and only I can be held responsible for any flaws and deficiencies this book may have.

–Angela Mailis-Gagnon, MD

I would like to thank my wife Susan Elliott, children Jacob, Tessa and Jemma for their patience, support and understanding of my work schedule. Thanks also to Reeve and Barbara Israelson and Clifford and Maxine Elliott for the many times they helped make that work schedule possible and to Bobby Rotenberg for being a good listener. In addition, thanks go—as ever—to Beverley Slopen, as well as the dedicated professionals at Viking; Nicole de Montbrun, Diane Turbide, Joe Zingrone, our superb copy editor Lisa Berland and Cynthia Good. Finally, I wish to acknowledge the support I have received from Patrick Gossage, my partners and the brilliant staff at Media Profile.

–David Israelson

Foreword

By Oliver Sacks

In April of 2002 I received an intriguing letter from a Dr. Mailis-Gagnon at Toronto Western Hospital. She said that she had founded a pain clinic there some 20 years before, and she spoke of a particular interest in patients who presented with severe pain, but then developed mysterious sensory or motor disturbances without any clear anatomical basis. Such disorders were usually dismissed as "functional" or "hysterical," but she and her colleagues had now found some of them to have a clear neurological basis. She was writing to me now, she said, because I seemed to have described a personal experience somewhat similar to this, in my book *A Leg to Stand On*.

I was excited by this letter; I had scarcely read two sentences, as I wrote to Dr. Mailis-Gagnon in my reply, before feeling, "Yes, that's it!" I had puzzled for more than a quarter of a century about my own experience (the original accident and nerve injury had occurred in 1974), without arriving at any clear conclusion. Moreover, there had been prior descriptions going right back to the Civil War of such strange sensory and motor disorders occurring in the wake of shock or pain—descriptions that were highly consistent, but inexplicable in terms of classical neurology or even psychiatry. And now, it seemed, Dr. Mailis-Gagnon might indeed, with a bold hypothesis and brilliant experiments, have provided an answer to the mystery.

Bringing to her work the patience and empathy of a dedicated physician and the incisiveness of a trained neuroscientist, Dr. Mailis-Gagnon, along with her colleagues, has revolutionized our understanding and treatment of chronic pain, doing for chronic pain what her mentor, the late Patrick Wall, did for acute pain (it was Wall, she mentioned in her original letter to me, who had alerted her to my book, when he visited Toronto in 1998). Over the years, Dr. Mailis-Gagnon has seen thousands of patients, patients for the most part referred to her by other physicians as hopeless or refractory cases. She has lectured to medical societies and published dozens of highly regarded papers on pain mechanisms, the genetics of pain, the epidemiology of chronic pain, etc., raising the medical awareness of these previously ignored areas. The proliferation of pain clinics in Canada and elsewhere bears witness to her pioneering efforts. And now, feeling a desire to distill the experience and thoughts of these 20 years, she has written a very vivid, very comprehensive and very personal book that is accessible equally to the general audience and the professional.

Wittgenstein once wrote that a book should consist of examples, and every chapter of *Beyond Pain* begins with clinical vignettes or case histories. We are introduced in chapter one to Costas and Chong Chi, in chapter two to Alex, in chapter three to Clara and Nicolette, and so on through a score of patients whose personalities and lives are presented as vividly as their pain. We come to know them as individuals, not as "cases," and their pains and other problems are not presented abstractly or medically, but in richly personal, nuanced, almost novelistic terms. There follows, in each chapter, a minute dissection of the pain mechanisms involved (the receptors, the anatomical pathways, the chemical mediators, and modifiers of pain, etc.), along with the secondary and tertiary reactions in the nervous system, if these occur (including the paralyses and anaesthesias that Dr. Mailis-Gagnon first wrote to me about). But most importantly—and it is this that is so rare, both in medical practice and in medical writing—Mailis-Gagnon explores the subjective experience of pain, its meanings and associations for each individual, its personal and social and cultural context. Thus pain (especially chronic pain) is seen as a behaviour, a total and sometimes very complex response, a creation of the individual person. Without such an approach, at once comprehensive and deeply personal, a so-called biopsychosocial approach, pain, at least in its more complex and chronic forms, may, as Dr. Mailis-Gagnon feels, remain unintelligible—and untreatable.

The range of topics covered in *Beyond Pain* is very wide, and one is likely to find almost any question about pain that one has ever puzzled over, explored somewhere within its pages. Why is there sometimes intense and very real pain despite seemingly minor injuries or provocations? Why, conversely, may very major injuries scarcely be felt? What mechanisms exist for blocking pain? Why is childbirth less painful than it might be? Why is the experience of pain, however intense, subsequently forgotten (or at least unrememberable) unless it occurs again, when it is instantly recognized? Why is pain less intense, or even unnoticed, in battle, conditions of great stress, or during vigorous exercise? What is the nature of "runner's high"? Why is sunburn so painful? Why do some people not respond to codeine? What is the proper use of opiates? What is the relation of pain to fear, depression or emotion in general? What did frontal lobotomies do to patients with intractable pain? Are there significant differences between men and women in their reactions to pain? What is "neuropathic" pain? What is reflex sympathetic dystrophy and causalgia? What is "central" pain? What is angina, referred pain, visceral pain? What is phantom pain—and how may it be treated? How do placebos, hypnosis, biofeedback and acupuncture work? What is going on with the current epidemic of low back pain, and of fibromyalgia, rheumatism and other allied conditions?

All this is treated here, and a dozen more topics, including Mailis-Gagnon's (and my) special interest—the nature of the mysterious "unanatomical" paralyses and anaesthesias that may follow in the wake of severe shock or pain. Mailis-Gagnon speaks of this as "functional de-afferentation," and she has shown, by the use of neuro-imaging, how the representation or map of the body in the sensory cortex may actually be "deactivated," shut down, at such times, as well as how such areas may be reactivated or opened up. Such work bridges the gap between "organic" and "functional," and shows the actual neural mechanisms involved in such "protective" or aberrant inhibitions. (This has important analogies to V. S. Ramachandran's remarkable studies with patients who have phantom pain, or inability to feel or claim parts of their own bodies in consequence of a stroke.)

And it testifies, like Ramachandran's work, and Merzenich's pioneer animal experiments, to the extraordinary plasticity of the nervous system, a plasticity undreamt of 20 years ago, and how this may work to a patient's advantage or disadvantage. Classical neurology pictures specific pain receptors in the skin and elsewhere, dedicated pain tracts in the spinal cord and specific receiving areas in

Costas, then 27, was the fourth of five siblings, three boys and two girls. His mother and father were born in a village in Northern Greece and had come to Montreal a few years earlier. Then they moved to Toronto, where they started their family after the father established a roofing business. Costas had dropped out of school in grade 10. He worked in his father's business and lived at home. Costas was fluent in English, as he was born in Canada, but his primary language at home was Greek.

When Costas entered my office I was impressed. He was unusually tall compared with the Greek men I knew and grew up with, maybe 1.9 metres (6 feet, 4 inches), slim, with intense but symmetrical facial features, beautiful big eyes and a large moustache. Truly a very attractive young man. We spoke half in Greek, half in English. Costas explained to me that he had slipped off a roof three years before, hit his chest on a beam and got a few bruises. Since that time he had intermittent pain in his chest. He did not think much of it and returned to work within a week. The government's workers' compensation scheme did not come into play, as Costas's father had not covered him with insurance. Despite returning to work, this chest pain appeared intermittently, lasting for a few minutes upon strenuous activity, including Costas's favourite pastime, weightlifting.

Costas had a well-equipped gym at home and used to work out at least five times per week. Both he and his family became increasingly worried about the chest pain. His general practitioner sent him to an orthopedic surgeon who diagnosed "subluxation of the sternomanubrial joint." I had never heard of this diagnosis before. The surgeon offered to "fix" it by fusing the joint. He said it was going to be a simple surgery, just two days in hospital. After discussing the issue with the whole family, Costas went for the surgery. Unfortunately, after the surgery Costas got worse, as his pain became almost constant. What bothered him more was a "grinding" he would feel over his chest bone on certain movements. Costas had not worked since the surgery. He abandoned his gym, his guitar and his friends. Desperate, the family sought other opinions. Costas ended up with another surgeon (the one who referred him to me), who told Costas that the first surgeon had not managed to stabilize the joint. He, as well, offered to "fix" it and assured Costas and his family that the solution would be permanent this time, as he was going to use wires. Unfortunately, 14 months and two surgeries later, Costas was in the same desperate position, with ongoing pain and grinding.

As Costas was giving me his history, he seemed to be in obvious distress. His beautiful face was twisted with pain, he walked slowly, stooped over, he was fidgeting in his chair and he sighed frequently. He was mourning the loss of his previous self, his gym, his guitar, his friends and his girlfriend who had left him, unable to cope with his chronic pain. When I asked him to rate his pain on a scale from 0 to 10, where 0 means no pain at all, and 10 is the worst pain ever, he told me that his pain during the history taking was 9. He added that when he moved around, the pain was as high as 15! In vain I tried to explain to him that level 10 would be enough to make one contemplate suicide. I could hardly make him move his arms or his neck, as he complained bitterly of chest pain. It was nearly impossible to touch Costas even gently over the sternum, as he would withdraw sharply. His overall presentation to me was coloured by "pain behaviours": intense expressions of pain both with words and body language. So, I decided, my only option was to admit him for a few days of investigation and assessment by my whole team, including the psychologist and the psychiatrist.

While Costas got admitted, I organized several tests. The first question I had related to Costas's surgery. Was the fusion he had undergone indeed solid? Did he have any physical source that was at least partially responsible for these complaints? In the meantime, he was to be seen by several members of my team.

During a four-day stay in the hospital, Costas chose to remain in bed, except when he had to go for tests. His pain ratings were very high even at rest. He always had visitors around him, brothers, sisters, his mom, dad, other relatives and friends. During our team rounds, the young psychology assistant, Cheryl, described Costas's behaviour when he became thirsty while completing some psychology questionnaires. As he bent over to drink from the fountain he would howl, to the point that psychology staff and other patients down the corridor became alarmed.

By the end of Costas's stay we had collected all the necessary test data and we met as a team. Traditionally, when we finish our discussion about the in-patients we have during a particular week, I visit each patient with my clinical fellow (a doctor training under my supervision to become a pain doctor) and other staff to let the patient know what the pain team concluded and what plans we had. I was not surprised to find out that Costas's fusion was not solid. Three investigations (tomograms of the sternum, a bone scan and a CAT scan) showed that the bones around the fusion were fragmented instead of being a solid mass. Furthermore, the wires were broken. No wonder Costas was feeling this grinding. So we had an answer as to the physical origin of Costas's complaints. But could the unstable fusion account for the profound degree of pain that Costas was enduring?

It was extremely unlikely. According to my team's psychiatrist and psychologist, Costas's pain had much deeper roots, in factors that were not physical. To be blunt, Costas had never really grown up. He was immature and extremely dependent and tended to express emotional conflicts as physical complaints. He also had a strong preoccupation with bodily functions and viewed his physique as one of his major assets, if not the greatest. Secure within a highly protective home environment, he never really had to work outside the family business. The traditional mesh of a closely knit Greek family, where grown-up children often remain at home indefinitely, was both Costas's support system and a detriment. For Costas, his injury and the subsequent failed surgeries meant that he could not rely any more on his physical prowess. He was left desperate and confused, with no answers as to what was wrong, or what was going to happen to him in the long run.

After the end of the rounds I walked with members of the team into Costas's room. He was waiting for me anxiously, surrounded by members of his family. I sat by the bedside.

"Costas," I said, "what do you want first, the bad news or the good news?"

He replied: "The bad news."

"Costas, I am afraid that you were right when you complained about this grinding sound in your chest. I am sorry, but your fusion is not solid despite what you were told. I also have to tell you that it is highly unlikely that the problem can be fixed by a third surgery."

"I knew it!" he shouted. "That bastard [his surgeon] was lying to me!"

"Now," I continued, "here comes the good news. Even if we would not recommend another surgery, we certainly think that you can get much better. Somewhere deep in your mind you thought that feeling pain with movement meant that you were going to cause more damage to yourself every time you wanted to be active. So you cut down on all your activities, you developed all kinds of guarding behaviours, like walking stooped, not moving much and so on, and naturally you became depressed. You started taking these strong painkillers but really they did nothing much to correct your problem or significantly help your pain. All of these feelings and behaviours can change. You will continue to hear this grinding sound from time to time, but you will probably get used to it. You can't get worse and if you avoid certain movements that bring significant pain, you will be all right. I will not promise you that you are going to be 100 per cent the way you were before, but I can assure you that you can be much better than what you are now and you can go on having a very good life."

I provided Costas and the family with the address of an outpatient cognitive-behavioural treatment program that I very much trusted. Unfortunately, the program was not covered by our government health insurance plan, and Costas's family would have to foot a substantial bill of several thousand Canadian dollars for a six-week outpatient program. His father assured me that money was not an issue. Costas was discharged home the same day.

Three months later, my secretary, Anna, paged me. It was Monday afternoon around 5:30 or 6:00. She said "a whole bunch of people" were waiting for me but would not tell her what they wanted. She did not recognize anyone. I finished seeing in-patients on the ward and returned to the office. In front of my office, four people were waiting for me. Vaguely I recalled the elderly couple. But . . . who was that tall, extremely good-looking fellow with the beard and an armful of roses?

"Hi Doc," he said.

It was Costas. I could not believe my eyes. The young man was standing tall, walking fast and freely into the room, with his shirt half open to the chest, strutting proudly in his designer jeans.

"You look awfully good," I said. "I had a hard time recognizing you."

"Well, you see, I finished the program you sent me to six weeks ago. It did me good, Doctor. I think I am getting back on track."

What had happened? Costas had attended the program with enthusiasm. He was taught how to reduce his pain by learning that "hurt" does not necessarily mean "harm," how to pace himself and to start restoring activities gradually. He had started training again in his home gym, he was jamming on his guitar regularly, he had gotten back into the groove of seeing his buddies and he was planning to try returning to his father's roofing business soon.

"Thank you, Doctor," he said. "I owe you and your team so much."

I never heard from Costas (or his surgeon) again. I am sure he is doing well. But I have used his case on numerous occasions to teach first-year medical students about the multiple dimensions of pain, and how mind over matter can make such a difference.

The experience of another patient, Chong Chi, was totally different—yet mind over matter played an equally important role. This fellow, 68 years old, was a wealthy Hong Kong businessman who had recently immigrated to Toronto with his family. He brought several million dollars with him. Chong Chi came to see me accompanied by his much younger, exquisitely dressed, wife, his son (whose cell phone never stopped ringing) and an interpreter. His primary complaint was a "minor neck ache," as the interpreter put it. "Oh yes, there is some numbness as well in the first three fingers of both hands but not much pain there."

On examination, I found that Chong Chi hardly moved his neck beyond a few degrees in each possible plane of movement. No matter how much he tried to co-operate or how much I pushed, I could not increase his range. He assured me with a gracious smile that he only felt "kind of stiff and a little achy, but nothing much." When I examined his deep tendon reflexes, I saw that he had lost the brachioradialis and triceps jerks—the reactions by these muscles to taps from the percussion or "reflex" hammer—in his left arm. There was also some specific muscle weakness. All of these were signs of nerve root damage. The nerve roots contain nerve fibres, and as they exit from the spinal cord, they form nerves, like the sciatic nerve at the back of the thigh or the median nerve in the arm and wrist, the one that is often pinched in carpal tunnel syndrome suffered by musicians, typists and pregnant women. The roots can be compressed as they exit from the cord by arthritic changes. If the compression is severe and extends to the spinal cord itself, the patient may end up with serious problems like paralysis or inability to control his bladder or bowels. I asked him whether he had any bowel or bladder problems and he said no.

At the end of my examination I was sure that on clinical grounds there was clear evidence of radiculopathy (compression of the nerve root by a prolapsed disk) involving some of the cervical roots that provide nerve supply to the arm. Fortunately, my patient had no signs or symptoms of spinal cord compression.

Chong Chi did not wish to go for any tests. Through the interpreter he informed me that he had taken acupuncture, but to no avail. He also said he had brought with him some "old" X-rays, since he did not want them repeated. My jaw dropped when I saw these old X-rays taken at least five years before.

What a mess! Every single disc space in his neck was extremely narrow. Thick bony protrusions (called osteophytes) were sticking out. The little holes from which the cervical roots exit from the bony canal, called foramina, were extremely narrow and I bet that several nerve roots were trapped and compressed. Given Chong Chi's resistance to further treatments or tests, I asked him what he expected of me. He replied that he thought, "Maybe . . . there was a pill to just decrease his discomfort a little."

I prescribed one of the newest Aspirin-like drugs. Perhaps it could help if there was some degree of inflammation within the joints.

I saw Chong Chi (and his family) six weeks later. He was a happy man. His range of movement had not changed one iota, his muscle weakness and wasting had not improved and his reflexes had not come back, but his subjective feelings of stiffness and discomfort were nearly gone.

Why did Costas and Chong Chi react so differently to pain and express their discomfort in such startlingly different ways? To understand their reactions, we need to explore how psychological factors and our cultural backgrounds influence our individual pain experience.

Illness Behaviour and Pain

The concept of illness behaviour is of paramount importance. It enables us to understand how people monitor their bodies, define and interpret their symptoms, see themselves as healthy or sick, take action and seek relief, by using traditional, lay or alternative sources of help.[1] But the concept of *illness* is very different from the concept of *disease*. A disease refers to a specific clinical entity associated with disturbed function or structure of a body part, organ or system. Illness, on the other hand, is a much wider concept, relating to the way we view sickness.[2] It reflects not only our psychological makeup but also the influences we receive from our socio-economic and cultural milieu.

The difference between disease and illness helps explain why some people with serious diseases go on with their lives, while others with minimal physical disorders may be highly disabled and feel ill—they display what we call "illness behaviour."

It is helpful to think of illness behaviour as a process of four elements interacting:[3] symptom perception, symptom interpretation, symptom expression and coping behaviours. Illness behaviour usually starts when some sign of change in our body is perceived as a sign of ill health. This perception occurs because we assign a meaning to what we feel. We base such assumptions on past experiences and a host of psychological and cultural factors. Assigning a meaning is important because it gives us some sense of understanding. For some patients this understanding may provide a sense of control and may also enhance their self-esteem. On the other hand, others may feel a sense of loss of control, while their self-esteem plummets. Whatever meaning we assign to these body signals will mobilize our attention. Pain in particular has the peculiar property of getting worse when we focus on it. The interpretation of symptoms and the meaning we assign to them varies tremendously between different groups or individuals and can profoundly affect the way we cope.

We express and communicate pain through both verbal and non-verbal behaviours, which involve body movements, postures, sighing, grimacing, rubbing, gasping and saying "Ouch!" and writhing. The forms of pain expression we use influence the way others judge our pain as well. As a matter of fact, those patients who tend to use extensive pain behaviours or expressions may be looked upon by others, including health providers, as "hyperreactive," "histrionic" or even "making it up." Others who behave in a stoic fashion may be taken more seriously by doctors, nurses and other health practitioners. What individuals express is not necessarily the same as what is happening to them. Some sufferers deny the symptoms, others exaggerate. Chronic pain, like any other chronic illness, will lead to the mobilization of coping mechanisms that may be adaptive or maladaptive—if you suffer you will try to cope, and it may work or it may not. Pain, the way we cope with it and how others perceive us is an intricate, rich mixture of what is going on inside us, how this is perceived by others and how the two interact—a blend of physical, emotional, psychological, social and cultural factors.

The Psychology of Pain

Because the last few decades have seen amazing advances in medicine, psychology and other fields of science, we are gradually shifting our attention away from merely "patching up" problems toward issues of chronicity (looking at how "chronic" problems arise and recur) and the maintenance of "wellness." With chronic pain, one of the major battles—only half won in my opinion—is the concept of mind versus body. The dichotomy has dominated our thinking for hundreds of years. This kind of dualism allows people to think that chronic pain may be either "real" or "imaginary." The concept of "imaginary" pain (also called "psychogenic" or "non-organic" pain) implies that pain may be exclusively generated by one's thoughts, imagination or psyche and may have no physical origin at all. Among pain practitioners the thinking is moving beyond this split. There is now growing agreement that pain, and in particular chronic pain, is multidimensional and that one must see the problem from its biological, psychological and social dimensions to get the whole picture. Even so, unfortunately, many doctors bound by conventional medical thinking still see things as caused by either mind or body.

Pain is ubiquitous, and it is also unavoidable. When it serves as a warning it is necessary. Pain is also a signal for us to adapt to the situation or do something about it. For example, the soreness and the burning of the skin after prolonged exposure to the sun may make us avoid or decrease our exposure to the sun's rays or use protective barriers like hats and sunscreens. But when pain becomes chronic and intractable, it can dominate a person's existence and lead to demoralization, distress and changes in the way one sees oneself. Pain may take over and become the governing force in the sufferer's life.

Chronic pain is a widespread problem. A Canadian study showed that at least 10 per cent of the population suffers from some form of persistent or frequently occurring pain.[4] Twenty-five per cent of the families surveyed said that at least one family member suffered from persistent pain. Another Canadian study found that 37 per cent of all patients visiting their family doctor complained of pain in the abdomen, chest, head or back, and for one-third, significant psychological factors accounted for their complaints.[5] Other Western countries are similar. It's important to remember, though, that patients who visit pain clinics like mine are not exactly representative of what goes on in the general population. Research confirms that patients attending pain clinics have significantly more psychosocial and adjustment problems associated with considerable disability than patients seen in the offices of family doctors.[6]

Many of us, as we get older, may suffer from long-lasting or recurrent pains. As long as we cope and life goes on, we just have "chronic pain." But when pain takes over our life, when sadness and hopelessness set in, then we suffer from "chronic pain disorder" or "chronic pain syndrome." It is this chronic pain syndrome/disorder that is harder to treat and requires a complex approach, addressing both the physical and emotional components of pain.

Chronic pain disorder can also be associated with mental disorders such as anxiety, depression and an array of so-called somatoform disorders, for example hypochondriasis, in which undue focus is placed on physical symptoms, and conversion disorder, in which emotional conflicts are expressed in physical problems. Several studies have shown a clear link between depression and chronic pain.[7] It's a vicious circle—chronic pain is more prevalent in patients with depression and depressed individuals complain of pain more. One would think that antidepressant drugs could help, but because the relationship between pain and depression is so complex, antidepressants work only on some patients with chronic pain, not everyone. Besides, there is no linear relationship between chronic pain and a particular personality. Chronic pain may provoke personality changes, create negative emotions and alter behaviour. But pre-existing personality traits such as irritability or intense preoccupation with physical symptoms may also magnify pain or prolong the pain after injuries.

But are there any circumstances where pain has *no physical origin* whatsoever, where it arises directly from emotions? This idea is central to the concept of hysteria (in which emotional stressors are expressed in physical symptoms such as blindness, paralysis and so on). One example of this type of situation is the couvade syndrome (from the French word for "hatching"), a phenomenon that has been well studied over the past 50 years. This syndrome is seen at childbirth in societies in Micronesia and the Amazon Valley.[8] The mother does not seem to suffer at all. She will take a few hours from working in the fields to give birth and then return back to her line of duty unhindered. But guess who suffers during childbirth? The husband lies in bed for several days and seems to be in agony, bewildered, groaning and moaning. The new mother, who never seemed to be in the slightest pain, sits by his side while he accepts congratulations from relatives who drop by! Of course, men do not have a uterus, so their pain would have to come from the mind.

As a concept, hysteria evolved over hundreds of years from the ancient times of Hippocrates, the father of modern medicine, to today. Sigmund Freud was the first to establish a psychological language for describing how body symptoms, including pain, may be the result of unresolved conflicts and troubled emotions, which in turn are converted and expressed in somatic complaints. Such a notion has been frequently employed to explain chronic pain symptoms when the doctors cannot find much wrong with a person's body. However, as science progresses and as our horizons widen, some symptoms and signs previously attributed to thoughts and emotions are found to have their roots in biology, including altered brain functions.

Disturbed thoughts are also known to be responsible for the experience or aggravation of pain. An example is a woman whose father died from stomach cancer, who herself experiences abdominal discomfort. Her first and most terrifying thought is that she has stomach cancer "exactly like her father." She agonizes over the idea and suffers with unbearable pain for days. Her physician orders some simple tests and she is assured that she has no cancer but a benign condition called irritable bowel syndrome. Once the assurance is given, her pain minimizes and becomes manageable, even without any medication or interventions.

Today, the modern approach to pain and psychological issues has shifted to emphasize an interactive process between thoughts and emotions, our bodies and our environment. Such concepts have led to the use of hypnosis and biofeedback techniques in pain management. Our ability to experience pain or create adaptive pain behaviours—for example when my right knee hurts, I will limp as I try to put less weight on this knee and for shorter periods of time— may depend also on learning processes through our growth and development.[9] It makes sense that a given behaviour will be repeated if there is a reward or reinforcement or it will cease if the reward is withdrawn. The technique of altering positive and negative reinforcements has been applied to chronic pain treatments in an effort to change pain behaviours.

Pain creates a private sense of hurt and a language to communicate this hurt.[10] This language involves behaviours and interactions, so pain also has a social context. When you have the flu there are associated symptoms and signs that go with it, so people around you know what you suffer from when they notice your fever, sneezing, facial flushing, sweats, pallid complexion and so on. But when your back hurts, there aren't necessarily visible signs . . . unless you show by your behaviour that you are in pain. You may limp, walk slowly or stooped, have difficulty getting out of your chair, sigh or verbalize pain or have facial expressions that show distress. All these are pain behaviours. These behaviours—verbal, as in saying, "Oh, my aching back," and non-verbal, as in stooping or grimacing—may or may not generate reactions from others. Those reactions and interactions—extra care or sympathy, doing things for you or, on the contrary, ignoring your pain—have been shown to exert powerful influences over the degree and duration of one's pain, particularly in a family environment. In particular, chronic pain in other family members, especially early in life, has been shown to influence strongly the degree and duration of one's pain in adult life.

One of the very first times I became fascinated with pain was at holiday gatherings with my parents' families while I was growing up in Greece. Mom came from a family of eight, four brothers and four sisters. Dad's family consisted of three brothers and three sisters. At our large family gatherings, Mom and her sisters and brothers would be quite busy comparing the number of doctor visits and the different medications they were given for arthritis, high blood pressure, cholesterol and God knows what. It was not unusual to hear complaints from one or another about the lower-quality care they had received if they were given fewer medications or felt deprived of the newer drugs that had come out. Meanwhile, Dad and his family never talked about pain or health issues. To the day of his death from lung cancer in 1980, I never heard Dad complain. Even when his voice was so hoarse that he could hardly be heard, he never once mentioned pain except for the odd discomfort because of his profound shortness of breath. Mom lived another 20 years after Dad's death. Until she became an invalid with dementia, I never spoke to her by phone without hearing her complain bitterly of different pains and other ailments, primarily her osteoarthritis. I kept reassuring her: "Mom, this form of arthritis will not kill you." I was quite right, as it was her heart that took her away at the age of 85 and not her joints. While the two sides of my family were so different in the way they expressed pain, my sister and I have both taken after my father's side when it comes to the perception of pain, our views of illness and the utilization of health care services (thank God for that!).

Other experiences and the meaning one attaches to pain also play a considerable role in shaping our perceptions. Soldiers severely wounded during the Second World War[11] or who suffered traumatic amputations in the 1973 Yom Kippur War[12] seemed to complain very little of pain or even not at all. The researchers who reported these astonishing behaviours felt that the primary reason was actually the meaning the soldiers attributed to their wounds: they had survived the battle, they were alive, and no matter what, they were going to be sent to hospitals far away from the battlefield to recuperate. The attribution of specific meanings that can change reactions to pain was shown much earlier in experimental animals. Early in the twentieth century, the famous scientist Ivan Pavlov experimented with dogs and showed that it was possible to alter the meaning of pain created by an electric shock to the point that the animals failed to feel much or any pain.[13] When a strong electric shock was given to one of the dog's paws, the dog seemed to hurt very much, react violently and withdraw its paw. However, when Pavlov presented a dish with food after each shock, the dogs developed a very different response. Instead of reacting strongly by moving away or barking, the dog would drool, wag its tail and run to the food. In other words, it had turned the electric shock from a signal of pain to a signal that food was on the way.

What about our attention? We all know that distraction can make us feel less pain. As a mother, I used to take my two boys to the doctor for their vaccines. I, like all other mothers, knew instinctively that giving the baby a sucker, a toy or a loud rattle would reduce his reactions and allow the nurse to deliver the injection more easily. In his wonderful book *Pain: The Gift Nobody Wants*, Dr. Paul Brandt[14] describes vividly how he managed to correct the distorted feet of newborns suffering from a disorder called talipes, better known as clubfoot, at the foot clinic of the Vellore Hospital in India after the Second World War. In this disorder, which affects newborns, one side of the foot is twisted, as the muscles, bones and ligaments are shorter on this side. The doctor had to apply gentle pressure to straighten the shortened side and stimulate it to grow without damaging the tissues. Then he would splint the foot in this position for five days, enough time to allow skin, ligaments and bones to adapt to the gentle stress and the new position. Each baby may need up to 20 castings of this sort, and then the feet are placed in splints until the baby starts walking. In this manner, the deformity gets corrected gradually. Dr. Brandt described how the waiting room "became a cacophony of squalling babies" because stretching and casting is a painful procedure. Ingeniously, he decided to shift the babies' attention away from the twisted foot while he was straightening it before he applied the cast, by introducing "an advanced state of hunger." In India mothers breast-feed their babies at least up to 12 months. All mothers were instructed to bring the babies to the clinic very hungry. As each mother was called with her infant, she sat opposite to the doctor, opened her sari and exposed a breast bulging with milk. While the baby was completely absorbed in sucking greedily at the breast, the doctor was able to remove the old splint, wash the foot, check its range of movement, stretching it gently by forcing it carefully to a new position and then cast it.

Whether it is pain experienced in the laboratory as part of an experiment or pain experienced in everyday life, distraction can diminish it or make it literally disappear. Some of the worst types of pains are those experienced by patients with brachial plexus avulsion. The nerve roots that form the brachial plexus, which provides sensation and movement to the arm, are detached from the spinal cord after some sort of serious trauma (for example, falling from a speeding motorcycle on an outstretched arm). While there are certain kinds of surgeries or medications that may help these unfortunate patients, it is well known that a very effective way to reduce their pain is simply to tell them to "concentrate on something they very much like."[15]

Pain includes sensation, affect (emotions) and cognition (thoughts). Yet it is common both for patients with chronic pain and for physicians (other than those who are quite familiar with chronic pain) to associate pain only with a physical entity, falling into the trap of dualism of body and mind. The search for the physical cause may become a major driving force both for the physician and the patient. Unfortunately, we tend to forget that pain creates strong emotions as well, such as anxiety, depression, resentment, anger, irritability and a compelling drive to seek relief or reassurance.[16] Depression by itself may lead to pain complaints to the point where sometimes patients suffer from many pain problems without acknowledging consciously that they are depressed. In this situation, called "masked depression," the pain complaints go away when the depression is treated.[17] Powerful emotions may profoundly enhance our perception of pain and have to be addressed on their own merit. Ignoring them and concentrating only on the physical sources of pain is not a good form of pain management.

Similarly, we should not ignore the cognitive dimension of pain—our thoughts and interpretations. When we think, what we are really doing is evaluating a given experience and assigning a meaning or an interpretation to it. In pain situations, our thoughts include assessments such as, "Where is the pain coming from?" "How serious is it?" "What is the cause?" "What may the consequences be of what I am feeling now?" Our thoughts and their content, our beliefs as to the meaning of pain, our sense of being able to control what happens to us, our expectations and our personal style of perceiving, interpreting and responding to an event all constitute the cognitive dimensions of the pain experience.

Ethnicity, Culture and Pain

Maryann Bates, a professor at the School of Education and Human Development at the State University of New York, studied pain patients of different ethnic backgrounds. Bates contends that culture reflects "the patterned ways that humans learn to think about and act in their world."[18] Culture involves learned and shared styles of thought and behaviour within the social structure of one's world. It is different from ethnicity, a distinction that is necessary to bear in mind. Ethnicity refers specifically to the sense of belonging in a particular social group within a larger cultural environment, whose members may share common traits such as religion, language or ancestry.

Studies on the relationship between ethnicity and pain can be problematic, but they can reveal implications for diagnosis or pain management that can be helpful, particularly when an ethnic group shares a common culture. For example, health care practitioners may find it useful to know that Hispanic cancer patients find religious faith a powerful resource in coping with pain, or that only 10 per cent of adult dental patients in China routinely receive local anaesthetic injections from their dentist for tooth drilling, compared with 99 per cent of adult patients in North America.[19]

The influence of culture and ethnicity on pain perception and expression has been a focus of research since the 1950s. It is true that ethnic groups may show distinct physiological and morphological characteristics. Examples of such characteristics are differences in the way certain drugs are metabolized,[20] or in muscle enzymes after exercise.[21] However, it is equally important to understand differences in pain perception and expression between ethnic groups, as these differences may have a bearing in diagnosis and management of pain. Indeed, both in the laboratory and in clinical settings, individuals belonging to different cultural or ethnic groups seem to react to or express pain differently. Research with adult twins supports the view that it is the cultural patterns of behaviour, not our genes, that determine how we will react to pain. As a matter of fact, culture may have a very early impact on reactivity to pain, even before the appearance of language.[22]

In a classic study, "old" Americans (white Anglo-Saxons whose families had been in the United States for several generations), Jews and Italians were shown to have different attitudes and expressions toward pain when tested in the laboratory.[23] The Anglo-Saxons faced pain stoically; they withdrew when pain was intense and cried out only when they were in solitude. While both Jews and Italians were very vocal in their complaints, the reasons for this were quite different: Jews were quite worried about the implications of persistent pain while Italians wanted a "quick fix." These differences have been duplicated in several other studies. All people, regardless of race or culture, seem to have the same "sensory perception thresholds" that signal our first awareness of a non-painful stimulus—tingling, warmth and the like. But our cultural background exerts a powerful effect on our threshold to feel pain, the "pain perception threshold." In an earlier, classic study, persons of Mediterranean origin described a form of radiant heat as "painful" while Northern European subjects called it simply "warm."[24]

A striking example of the influence of our cultural background on pain tolerance was shown in a study of subjects of different ethnic origin who had been given electric shocks. Women of Italian descent tolerated less shock than women of Anglo-Saxon or Jewish origin.[25] Interestingly, in another study, when women of Jewish and Protestant descent were told that their respective religious group had not done well compared with others, only Jewish women were able to tolerate a higher level of shock. These were the women who generally tolerated lower levels of shocks to start with. Since their cultural background was associated with earlier vocalization and complaints about pain, they had "more room to move" in terms of additional shock stimulus.[26]

In one study, the researchers tested six ethnic groups—"old" American, Hispanic, Irish, Italian, French Canadian and Polish subjects.[27] The Hispanics reported the highest pain levels and most of them had an "external locus of control." This term refers to cognitive perceptions or expectations regarding life events and circumstances, including illness and pain. A person with an internal locus of control feels that life events are the result of one's own actions. To the contrary, a person with an external locus of control feels that life events are outside his or her control and reside in the hands of fate, chance or other people.[28] In Maryann Bates's study, those pain patients who had an internal locus of control had much less work disruption, unhappiness, worry, fear or depression.

In yet another study, patients in a pain centre in New England were compared with those in an outpatient medical centre in Puerto Rico. The Puerto Ricans (Hispanics or Latinos) were found to experience higher-intensity pain, a finding that supports the long-held belief that Latino cultures are more reactive to pain. However, when Puerto Ricans who had immigrated and lived in New England for several years were tested, their reactions were more similar to those of the New England group than their original Puerto Rican group. Obviously, the pain responses of people from different ethnic groups can change, as they are shaped and reshaped by the culture in which the people live or move into.[29]

An extreme example of cultural influences in the perception and expression of pain is the procedure of "trepanation" in East Africa.[30] This is a surgery for which men and women do not get any anaesthetics or any painkilling drugs. The *doktari* (tribal doctor) cuts the muscles of the head to uncover the bony skull. Then he scrapes it while the patient sits calmly, fully awake, and holds a pan to collect the dripping blood! He or she does not flinch, does not withdraw, does not show a hint of distress but assists in the surgery. It is the Westerners viewing videotapes of the procedure who feel extreme distress as their stomachs turn. We will see these and even more remarkable attitudes to pain when we discuss in coming chapters how certain cultures actually block the pain in gruesome rituals or initiations.

While understanding the impact of culture and ethnicity in pain expression is important, ethnic differences between patients and medical professionals may lead to dangerous consequences. For example, different studies have shown that patients of certain ethnic backgrounds (Asian, black and Hispanic) are less likely than whites to receive adequate analgesia in the emergency room or be prescribed certain amounts of powerful painkilling drugs such as opioids.[31] Researchers have also determined that some pharmacies in non-white neighbourhoods of New York City stock inadequate supplies of opioids for the treatment of severe pain compared with pharmacies in white neighbourhoods.[32] Worldwide differences in administration of opioids in non-white nations are not, however, solely due to medical decision-making but may relate to politics. For example, it has been shown that the U.S. campaign against drug trafficking may account for the inadequate pain relief available to cancer patients in Mexico.[33]

Paying too much attention to ethnic behavioural and perceptual differences can also cloud and obscure similarities. The challenge is to understand not only how the human experience of pain includes differences between specific groups, but also similarities that bind us together, despite our diverse and changing backgrounds.

Understanding My Patients

Let's attempt now to interpret the experiences of Costas and Chong Chi. In Costas's case, his intensely expressive "language of pain" led him to display his distress with many and remarkable pain behaviours. Expressing emotions in strong ways through both verbal expressions and body language is integral to Mediterranean and other cultures. Costas's pain behaviours led to reactions of sympathy, offers of help and support by the members of his closely knit family. His personal distress was immense. Scientists use the word "pain" to describe the sensory experience associated with something harmful or potentially harmful, while the term "suffering" is reserved to describe "our emotional reaction to a noxious stimulus." The emotional distress may be quite disproportionate to the actual intensity of the sensory experience. Costas "suffered" from intense pain and displayed it loudly. He did not know what was wrong with him, why he was still feeling pain or whether he was ever going to get better. The thought that his physical prowess was not there and that he had no idea if it was ever going to be restored was demoralizing. Costas had lost control over his life—and his pain.

Obviously, Costas's encounters with my team changed his perception of pain. We did nothing to alter the physical cause of his pain, but we did a lot to change his suffering. What seemed to change in him were his beliefs, expectations and coping mechanisms. In the first place, what I thought was bad news (that his fusion was not solid and that he should not go for another surgery), became good news for him. In his mind, the discovery of the broken fusion had truly vindicated him. He became convinced that the grinding he was feeling all along was real and not a figment of his imagination. Besides, he did not want to go for more surgery (or as he later told me, to see any more doctors). The team's recommendation against additional surgical intervention suited him fine. He was told that he can lead a near-normal life and that he won't get worse. Once Costas had an explanation of the underlying cause and was given guidance as to the avenues of treatment available to him, his sense of despair, fear, anger, irritability and hopelessness changed. Furthermore, by attending the cognitive-behavioural pain program I sent him to, his beliefs about the meaning and interpretation of his pain changed and he felt he could have more control over his life. He continued to complain of local tenderness if one was to press hard on the sternomanubrial joint, as well as of his familiar grinding sound. But he could cope with these signs now as he knew where they were coming from and what they meant.

On the other hand, Chong Chi had always learned to restrain his emotions. He had a tremendous amount of degenerative changes in his neck (what we call arthritis), but his pain tolerance was high, his expressions of discomfort extremely

light the swelling in Alex's finger looked angry and in full bloom, and, like most three-year-olds in such circumstances, he wouldn't stay still. "Hurt!" he cried, and he ran away from the sink. I panicked. There was no one else at home, it was late, Nicholas was asleep and that finger was only going to get more and more swollen. I called my next-door neighbour and asked him if he would mind watching his TV show in my living room so I could leave quickly for the nearest hospital emergency. I hurried there and even at 10:30 p.m., the emergency room was packed. It was a microcosm of contemporary society, with the added dimension of sick-room anxiety—the nervous faces of young and old, trendy and stolid, rich and poor of all backgrounds, with Alex and me blending in.

Despite his predicament, Alex cruised the room curiously, exploring all the other people who were waiting to be called. From time to time he would show others his swollen index finger, and then he would sit down to play with some spare blocks lying on the floor. Although he was the reason for our being there, he seemed comfortable most of the time. I certainly was not. His finger looked more and more swollen, the normal creases of skin were gone and the entire digit had a rather purplish colour. "No good," I was thinking. It was already an hour and I had approached Alex a couple of times to check the finger. He seemed quite absorbed with the blocks and only when I inquired, he would say "burn, squeeze." I asked the nurse impatiently when Alex was going to be seen and received a brisk response—there were many other people before him. . . . I called home to speak to my neighbour and found out that my then-husband had returned unexpectedly. I explained to him what happened and how we were waiting. He urged me to return home, because "maybe all of us can try to take this thing out." That seemed at least possible, since on my own I had failed to immobilize a three-year-old.

By midnight, when I parked the car in the driveway, Alex ran to the house to show his dad the "big finger." It had reached the point where there was not much time for talk. My neighbour, a tall man, gave Alex a headlock while I threw my whole body into an embrace around my son's little legs. This did not save me from a few good kicks, yet while Alex became totally consumed in an effort to escape, his dad rubbed some vegetable oil around the swollen finger and within few seconds he pulled the nut off. I could not tell who was sweatier at the end, the tiny boy with his newly freed finger or the three adults who had been so worried about the consequences of persisting constriction on his hand.

There was a visible mark at the base of Alex's swollen finger, but the colour was quickly returning to normal. Yet once the nut was removed, Alex howled. "Burn," he cried, screaming and squirming incessantly, waving his hand wildly, in sharp contrast to his calm activity during our wait at the emergency room. I tried to console him but he refused to go to bed and would not allow me to touch the finger. Finally, he demanded to "see Ninja," the group of four martial art turtle warriors that had just come out in the market. It was early into the next day already, so I gave in easily. The Ninjas did their magic. Within five minutes Alex was profoundly asleep. The next morning he described his finger as "bit burning," but only if squeezed hard or if he was asked. The day after, everything seemed to have been forgotten—at least for him.

As a mother, you never forget these events. As a doctor and researcher, I understood in all too vivid detail where Alex's physical pain had come from. The tight nut around his finger was creating a condition called ischemia, which happens when a part of the body suffers a lack of blood supply. This condition led to the production of certain substances that stimulated nerve endings within the finger, which in turn sent the danger signal to Alex's brain.

You don't need to be an expert to understand that relationship—the tight nut around the finger causes constriction leading to loss of blood supply to the muscles, nerves and bones and creates pain. But was the stimulation to the nerve endings by irritating substances secreted during ischemia all that was needed to make Alex "feel" pain? Something didn't add up. Why did Alex seem oblivious to the increasingly swollen finger when he was busy playing with the blocks in the emergency room, and why did he keep screaming after the nut was removed?

Maybe we can better understand what Alex was feeling if we try to define exactly what "pain" is. But that's not easy. There are no human beings who have never felt pain, except some very rare exceptions whom we will meet later in this book. Despite the fact that pain is a universally encountered experience, there are many, many definitions of pain. For the scientist, pain is the result of stimulation of nerve endings by a harmful stimulus—pinch, pull, stretch, strong heat, acid and so on. For others, the word pain refers to the emotional reaction of the individual to the stimulus the body perceives as harmful. This emotional reaction reflects one aspect of our suffering. Overall, the term "pain" has come to have a different meaning for the scientist, the psychologist, the priest, the lawyer, the philosopher, the office worker, the politician or the one who feels the pain.

The International Association for the Study of Pain (IASP) has adopted the definition proposed by the internationally known Canadian psychiatrist, Dr. Harold Merskey: "Pain is an unpleasant sensory and emotional experience associated with actual or potential tissue damage, or described in terms of such damage."[1] This definition accepts that pain is a subjective experience that has both "sensory" dimensions (as they relate to damaged tissues) and "affective-cognitive" dimensions (the experience is associated with emotions and thoughts). This definition is widely accepted by those who research and treat pain, but it is far from being all-encompassing and will not satisfy everyone all the time.

When we experience pain, say from an acute back strain, a kidney stone or an inflamed tooth, most of us become pain-free once the disorder that produces it goes away. Yet a small but significant number of people develop long-lasting, chronic pain. Are they just unlucky? Are they complainers? We all know such people but we don't understand well what differentiates those who become chronic pain patients from those whose pain goes away. While we may understand much about the science of pain, even today we know very little about some of the most common clinical problems, for example, low back pain. Who among us has reached middle age and not experienced low back pain? Yet the causes—physical, psychological and socio-environmental (a mixture of experience and surroundings)—can be so many and complex that even scientists do not have a solid understanding of all types and forms of this common problem.

Besides, there is no clear relationship between the amount of tissue damage and the degree of pain one experiences or the impairment of function one has. We know, though, that underlying psychological factors such as depression or anxiety do have an impact on the journey from acute pain to chronic pain and disability. To get anywhere close to understanding how chronic pain develops and is maintained, we must first explore how acute pain is created and perceived—what happens when hammer strikes thumb and the person at the end of that thumb shouts "Ouch!" Knowing how acute pain is generated can help with understanding how it is transformed into chronic, unrelenting pain.

Let's take an example of acute pain. When the sharp blade of a knife pushes lightly on our skin, we feel only pressure. However, harder contact with our skin will produce a cut or laceration; that indicates tissue damage. The sensation of pressure then will be transformed into sharp pain. What's happening is that the cut produced by the knife blade activates specialized "nociceptive neurons"—nerve cells that respond to noxious or potentially harmful stimuli. In most cases, tissue damage will simultaneously produce unpleasant feelings of worry, anxiety, aversion and others, and only then will it be perceived as pain. It is important to recognize that unless the nociceptive stimuli are associated with the unpleasantness, we do not really feel much pain. In the example of my son, it seems that Alex did not really associate the constrictive effect of the nut with unpleasantness when he was busy playing with the blocks. This probably happened because he did not really understand that his finger was going to be damaged if the ischemia were to last for long, and because he was displacing his attention from the finger to the toys.

The split between unpleasantness and noxious or harmful sensation has been noticed in studies of hypnotized individuals, who report intense heat sensations but no unpleasantness and do not complain of pain during hypnosis. Once they recover from their "altered" state of mind, they associate unpleasantness with harm and the same experiment generates a lot of pain. The unpleasant dimensions of pain are multiple and may include feelings such as anger, fear, despair and panic. Alex was only truly hurting when he brought into the picture these types of feelings, and whatever else he had in his heart with these three "big people" overtaking him, even though the constriction of the finger was gone and his circulation was restored.

To me, this story, so close to home, shows how difficult it is to produce an all-encompassing definition of pain. Pain truly represents a whole group of experiences with different causes, unique circumstances and different qualities.

Understanding the Science of Pain

Pain is part of a defence system responsible for warning the body of influences that may harm it, so that the body can mount a response. The warning signals are perceived by the body through specialized structures called receptors.

These receptors will recognize many kinds of warning signals, while the body will respond to these signals in several ways.

For example, a foreign body in your throat will produce a tickling sensation and an urge to cough. A foreign body in your eye will generate an uncomfortable sensation, which will make you blink and cause your eye to water in an effort to get rid of this irritation. An injury that may damage living tissues will create pain and the body will attempt to do something to avoid this situation. If you take a pan out of the oven and accidentally touch the hot metal edge, you'll pull your hand away quickly.

Scientists today accept that specialized neural pathways carry the sensations of seeing, hearing and taste. The physical stimulus—a glittering light, the slamming of a door, the mouth-watering sweetness of a dessert—activates specialized sensory nerve endings, gets carried by certain nerve fibres, and is processed in different regions of the nervous system, each specific to the particular sensation.

Is this also true for pain? Is pain truly "hard-wired" with specialized receptors, specialized neural pathways and dedicated central structures, exclusively devoted to perceiving just pain? The answer is not entirely clear—literally, it's yes and no. Pain has much in common with sensory experiences such as hearing and seeing, but it also differs in significant ways. Indeed, there are specific pain receptors; the messages generated by noxious stimuli travel to the spinal cord via specific nerves, and from there through specific pathways to higher brain centres.

But things are more complex than that. The processing of pain-related information involves four major steps. The first step is transduction—the receptors (nerve endings) are activated by tissue-damaging stimuli. The second step is transmission—the message is carried from the receptors to the brain through special fibres. The third step is modulation—a process that changes the activity in the transmission system. The final step is the perception of pain—the subjective awareness produced by sensory signals, which requires their integration as a meaningful whole. Perception is influenced and modulated by many complex functions such as attention, expectation and interpretation of the signals based on previous experiences and current thoughts.[2] In the end, "all pain is in the brain," which becomes clear when we follow these processes step by step.

Imagine again that you are cooking something in the oven. When the food is ready, you attempt to take the hot tray by holding it with a kitchen towel wrapped around your fingers. The towel slips . . . your fingertips touch the hot pan. Immediately you withdraw your hands from the hot surface in pain.

During these split seconds many things occur in your nervous system from the tip of your fingers to your conscious brain. Let's trace the steps.

Wiring

The diagram on page 28 shows the major pain pathways, where they start and how they end up in the brain. Referring often to this drawing will help understanding of the processes described in this section.

The hot pan contact generates a noxious (harmful) stimulus that activates the receptors of the nerves that supply the skin of your fingers. These receptors are involved in the process of signal transduction, as we discussed above. Once those skin receptors are activated, they will deliver a pattern of electrical impulses to the spinal cord via many nerve fibres at different speeds (transmission of signals). Nerve fibres look like individual strands, and bunches of them are contained in nerves—for example, the sciatic nerve that runs along the back of our thighs and that often gets pinched when we have a herniated disc. Pain-related impulses are conveyed through two kinds of slim pain fibres, called A-delta and C, which travel in the dorsal or posterior roots of the spinal cord that terminate at the dorsal horns (the upper parts of a butterfly-like structure along the whole length of the spinal cord). On the other hand, pain signals from internal organs such as the kidney or the stomach will travel to the spinal cord via different kinds of slim fibres, again joining the dorsal or posterior roots.

In the dorsal horns of the spinal cord, the electrical signals pass through a densely populated area of nerve cells, where not only do fibre connections occur but the signals coming from the skin of your finger can be changed or modified. A new set of fibres, which take the pain-related information from the spinal cord to the brain, arise from clusters of nerve cells within the dorsal horns. Close to their site of origin within the dorsal horns, these nerve fibres cross to the opposite side and ascend centrally via the spinothalamic tract, as the diagram shows. The spinothalamic tract has received a lot of attention because

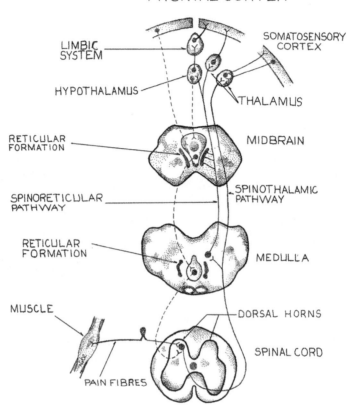

FRONTAL CORTEX

LIMBIC SYSTEM

SOMATOSENSORY CORTEX

HYPOTHALAMUS

THALAMUS

RETICULAR FORMATION

MIDBRAIN

SPINORETICULAR PATHWAY

SPINOTHALAMIC PATHWAY

RETICULAR FORMATION

MEDULLA

MUSCLE

DORSAL HORNS

SPINAL CORD

PAIN FIBRES

The pain pathways and their connections in the spinal cord and the brain. A tear in the muscle fibres (bottom left) stimulates specialized muscle receptors (nociceptors) and sends the message to the dorsal horns of the spinal cord via pain fibres. These fibres in turn connect with specialized dorsal horn cells that send pain signals to the brain via two pain pathways: The spinothalamic tract passes all the way through the lower part of the brain (medulla and midbrain) to specialized structures in the thalamus, ending in a specific part of the cortex, the somatosensory cortex, where the intensity and location of pain is recognized. The second important pain pathway is the spinoreticular tract that starts from the spinal cord and ends at the reticular formation, a cluster of nervous tissue within parts of the lower brain, including the medulla and the midbrain. Information from the spinoreticular pathway and the reticular formation continues to different areas of the thalamus and fans out to large regions of the brain, including the hypothalamus and other parts of the limbic system, which influence the emotions associated with pain. Connections from there to the frontal lobes make pain consciously recognized. The dotted line shows descending influences from different parts of the nervous system that change pain signals at multiple levels (process of modulation).

a person stops feeling pain when surgeons cut this tract at certain levels of the spinal cord. This tract ends at the thalamus, a very important structure within the brain that serves as a major connection node. The second important pathway for pain is the spinoreticular tract. It originates from many of the same nerve cell clusters as the spinothalamic tract, but also from other areas of the spinal cord. Its fibres reach the reticular formation, a cluster of nerve cells within the lower part of the brain stem (medulla and midbrain). The reticular formation plays an important role in alertness, generation of movements and behaviours that make us escape from unpleasant or harmful situations.

Subsequently, the information that arrives in specific parts of the thalamus via the spinothalamic tract is transmitted directly to a specific area of the cortex (the outer layer of the brain), called the somatosensory cortex, where the intensity and location of the pain is appreciated ("Hey, my finger hurts!"). On the other hand, information that arrives in certain other areas of the thalamus from the spinoreticular tract and the reticular formation will fan out in widespread projections to different areas of the brain, including the limbic system, which consists of several structures (hypothalamus, hippocampus, etc.). The limbic system influences the emotions and behaviours associated with pain. Some of the information from the thalamus and the reticular formation will also terminate in the frontal lobes (situated in the front part of the brain), where pain is consciously recognized. These pain signals, which by now have reached the brain all the way from the finger, have been much changed, as descending pathways send multiple influences throughout the nervous system, including the dorsal horns in the spinal cord (this is the process of modulation). Finally, pain will be perceived as such through the integration of many complex functions involving attention (you notice something hurts), previous experiences (you know you'll get a blister) and so on.

The Chemistry of Pain

Our knowledge of pain mechanisms has increased dramatically over the last several years. Chemical substances within the body are involved in both pain control and pain signals. Knowing the chemistry of pain is important because it allows us to use drugs with specific actions to treat specific problems, for example, inflammation. We have become better in our ability to pinpoint which drug will react with which particular substance. For example, substances involved in inflammation include histamine, serotonin and metabolites of arachidonic acid—prostaglandins and leukotrienes. Aspirin, one of the most common drugs, has many functions, but we now know that one of the most significant ones is its ability to reduce the swelling, heat and pain coming from an inflamed joint by inhibiting prostaglandin synthesis.

Many chemical substances simply block pain signals; others generate them. During the 1950s, many discoveries were made about *ascending* pain pathways and the chemicals that help the transmission of pain signals upward. Examples of chemicals that generate pain signals are substance P, vasoactive intestinal peptide and cholecystokinin, which are found in many areas of the nervous system. When it comes to chemicals that block the pain, the powerful analgesic (painkilling) effect of the poppy and the family of substances derived from it (opium, heroin and morphine) have been known for centuries. In the 1970s, researchers found out that some nerve cells have specialized receptors (opiate receptors) that bind to morphine. The scientists, of course, questioned why the body would have such a capacity to bind to morphine, since few of us go around using the drug constantly. Could it be because the body may have its own internal morphines?[3]

This line of thinking led to the discovery of morphine-like substances produced internally in the body—the body's own natural painkillers, or *endogenous opioids*. The discovery of these chemicals (enkephalins and endorphins) created a revolution in understanding and managing pain. These endogenous opioids, which are released from the nerve cells of the peripheral and the central nervous system, play a crucial role in the body's pain system. These chemicals operate within a distinct *descending* network that controls and modifies pain transmission. It is this network that is partially responsible for the dramatic variation of pain experienced by different patients, even though these patients may have the same type or degree of injury. Importantly, beyond controlling pain, they also exert a powerful effect on mood and sense of well-being.[4] However, the body's own internal opioids are not the only types of chemicals involved in modifying pain transmission. Scientists have discovered other endogenous substances (examples of which are epinephrine/norepinephrine and cannabinoids) that are important in pain modulation. I will discuss some of these substances in later chapters.

There are several situations that will trigger the release of endogenous opioids in our bodies, examples of which are brain stimulation, counterirritation, acupuncture, stress-induced analgesia and analgesia produced by vaginal stimulation.[5] About 30 years ago, researchers reported the use of electrical stimulation in a part of the brain called "periventricular grey matter" to treat patients with intractable pain. Most of the studies were done between 1973 and 1983. This technique is used sparingly now to treat serious pain problems when all other avenues of treatment have been exhausted (for example, in intractable pain after a stroke). This form of stimulation-produced analgesia has been shown to be mediated at least partially through the release of endogenous opioids.

Counterirritation has been known since antiquity. With this technique certain pains are alleviated by inflicting another acute pain. An ancient popular technique used to control pain, acupuncture, is a form of counterirritation. Studies of acupuncture consistently show that part of its effect is mediated through endogenous opioids.

Stress analgesia is related to counterirritation but is not identical. Stress can be either physical or psychological, resulting from surgery, labour, childbirth, stressful emotional states, chronic pain and so on. Vigorous exercise is also a known stress-inducer for the body. Again, the release of endogenous opioids has been shown consistently in several studies to account for the decrease in perceived pain. (This helps explain why a competitive football player who seriously injures his ankle may not feel the pain during the heat of the game.) These same internal painkillers are responsible for "runners' high," as endogenous opioids also affect our behaviours and sense of well-being.

Another fascinating topic specific to females and reproduction relates to analgesia occurring during vaginal stimulation. When several laboratories working with both animals and humans confirmed the existence of such analgesia, the researchers started wondering if this represented another form of stress-induced analgesia. The answer is yes, but only if we accept that stress does not have to be aversive but also can be pleasurable. Heart rate and blood pressure double during a woman's orgasm. So, from the physiological point of view, this is indeed a high level of stress for the body as the sympathetic nervous system, part of the autonomic nervous system, is highly activated. Yet the experience is intensely pleasurable.

Pain and Genes

Now, let's talk about another biological factor that may determine if and how much we hurt: our genes, which carry the blueprints of our identity and are located on our chromosomes. The chromosomes are structures within the nucleus of each cell in our body, composed of a linear thread of a specific acid called DNA (deoxyribonucleic acid), which carries our genetic material expressed in the form of genes. Mammals have 23 pairs of chromosomes with anywhere between 50,000 to 150,000 genes located on them. Variants of the genes (called alleles) contribute to the expression of our physical and other characteristics. They are what make us individuals. Genes determine how tall or short we are, the colour of our hair and eyes, the structure of our bodies, as well as behaviours and whatever abilities or disabilities we may have. Of course, the influence of our environment on the expression of genes is also a major factor. Very few traits or characteristics are controlled by a single gene. Most traits are shaped by multiple genes.

Many of the newest breakthroughs in the science of pain have occurred in the field of pain genetics, which is in its infancy compared with other fields. Significant progress has been made only in the last 20 years. Scientists now can look directly onto the material of genes and manipulate it, or study inherited variations or differences between members of the same species. For example, in humans, considerable differences have been documented between different individuals when it comes to pain sensitivity, response to different analgesics or development of certain pain syndromes.[6]

In people, few mutations (alterations) of single identifiable genes have been associated with pain-related disorders. In a rare inherited form of "insensitivity" to pain, researchers identified three single gene mutations affecting a specific set of neurochemicals and enzymes that regulate small pain fibres.[7] Another defective gene has been recognized in a rare inherited type of migraine (familial hemiplegic migraine).[8] But these isolated defective genes affect very small numbers of people. The only known pain-related gene that affects a large proportion of humans relates to the coding of a particular enzyme (P450IID6) that is responsible for the metabolism of at least 40 widely used drugs, including the powerful analgesic codeine. This defective gene that results in a non-functional enzyme exists in 7 to 10 per cent of all Caucasians. Since the individuals who carry this gene are unable to convert codeine into morphine, they may consume large quantities of this drug but it will not result in any pain relief.[9]

Most traits, whether pain or other characteristics and functions of our body, are usually mediated through multiple genes. This makes things much more difficult when we try to determine exactly which genes control a particular trait and where they are located in the vast territory of different chromosomes. When it comes to the heritability of pain arising specifically from lesions of the nervous system, the first evidence for genetic transmission was described in rats by the team of my colleague Marshall Devor from Jerusalem.[10] But when it comes to people with pain from nervous system damage, a little study I did with my colleague Judy Wade back in the early 1990s was the first to suggest that women with a particular neuropathic pain syndrome (reflex sympathetic dystrophy) had some markers indicating that perhaps they were genetically vulnerable to developing this syndrome.[11] Five years later, our results were duplicated by another group of researchers in the Netherlands.[12] Since then, Judy Wade and I have looked at the same type of clinical syndrome with more detailed blood analysis (this time trying to apply DNA-based techniques) in an attempt to come closer to the culprit genetic markers.[13] Other researchers around the world are also looking for possible genetic associations in humans with other pain syndromes like phantom limb pain and post-mastectomy syndrome.

There is no doubt that such pain genes exist. But environmental and psychosocial conditions do strongly influence gene expression; both "nature" and "nurture" are powerful forces, interacting in many ways. There is a lot of popular speculation today that, thanks to the recent mapping of the human genome, we will all someday walk around with gene maps, perhaps imprinted on cards, to determine what kind of medical treatment would work best in given situations. But except in situations relating to our ability to respond to certain drugs, I feel it is highly unlikely that gene maps alone will determine what forms of treatment we should or should not receive to combat different kinds of pains. The influence of our thoughts and our environment more frequently than not override Mother Nature—what we think and experience can't be predetermined on a little computer card or a Medic-Alert bracelet.

The Feeling of Pain

So, after you touch a hot pan, how do you end up feeling pain? Actually you will feel two types of pain, one after the other within milliseconds. The first pain is felt instantly as a sharp, well-localized sensation in your fingertip at the site of the burn. The second one feels like a dull, throbbing or burning sensation that involves diffusely the whole finger, and persists longer, perhaps for several minutes. The first pain is conducted through pain fibres that transmit information fairly fast, the A-delta pain fibres that will help you to precisely localize the pain. The other type of dull, aching, burning pain is transmitted via a slower-conducting type of nerve fibre—these are the C fibres, which generate a more disagreeable and persistent type of pain. Most acute clinical problems involve a mixture of both types of pain. It has been shown that the strength and duration of the pain carried by the C fibres may be affected by age and sex and is different in patients with fibromyalgia (a painful soft tissue disorder) and temporo-mandibular disorder (painful affliction of jaws and surrounding tissues) when compared with normal people.[14]

But beyond types of pains and pain fibres, pain is shaped by the brain as a whole. Every single brain activity—all five senses—may contribute to our perception of pain, including simply thinking. To consciously perceive pain, many areas of the brain must function in a dynamic interplay. The reticular formation drives us to avoid a painful or unpleasant stimulus. The limbic system plays a major role in aversive behaviour and in colouring our experiences with emotions. The specific areas of the thalamus where the spinothalamic tract ends contain a mini-map of the human body and allow us to discriminate a stimulus and determine its origin. Other parts of the thalamus that do not have this mini-map ability are connected to emotions and aversive behaviours through links with the reticular formation and the limbic system, as we discussed earlier.

The cortex (the outer "shell" of the brain) also plays multiple roles in pain perception. Part of the cortex, called the primary somatosensory cortex, will localize and identify the sensory input. This input can then be compared to previous experiences and assessed properly, so a decision can be made to take one or another course of action. However, different connections between many cortical regions will involve our memory, attention, previous experiences and all kinds of feelings.

The importance of emotions in colouring our pain experience can better be understood by the behaviour of patients who have undergone a neurosurgical procedure called frontal lobotomy. The frontal lobes of the brain play an important role in many cognitive activities and emotions. A frontal lobotomy severs the connections between the frontal lobes and the thalamus. This surgery was popular after the First World War to treat amputees with a special kind of agonizing pain, phantom limb pain, in which a person feels pain at the site of an amputated limb. Frontal lobotomies were popular particularly in the United States, where more than 50,000 are believed to have been performed. People who were subjected to this procedure were still able to localize the pain but they would say they didn't care. That means that the emotional colouring of the pain, the unpleasantness, the anguish and the avoidance behaviour to escape pain were minimized, while the ability to localize pain remained. Unfortunately, these patients also experienced dramatic personality changes. The surgery was eventually abandoned, but the unwanted effects encountered by patients subjected to it show us the immense dangers of premature application of medical knowledge.[15]

To put all this together, once the information is in the brain, the brain will help localize the source of pain, initiate rapid protective measures (for example, withdrawal of your finger—the motor component), raise your blood pressure, make you sweat, generate deep breathing or heart palpitations (the autonomic component), and evoke emotions and colour your pain experience based on previous memories and current thoughts. It is important to remember that getting the signals from the finger to consciousness is not a simple one-way street. Throughout this whole sequence, the signals generated at your fingertips will be changed in multiple ways and lead you to avoid touching the hot pan. Most signals start as "harm" signals and may or may not be translated into pain or "hurt" signals by the time they reach the conscious brain.

The late Dr. Patrick Wall, a legendary guru of pain, was the co-founder of the "gate control" theory in the mid-1960s.[16] Together with Ronald Melzack, a renowned Canadian neuroscientist and psychologist from McGill University, he developed the concept that pain signals coming from the periphery (skin, muscles, joints or internal body organs) are changed and influenced by non-pain signals coming upward from body parts or downward from the brain and other structures of the nervous system (refer back to the diagram on page 28). This conceptual framework of the modulation of pain was revolutionary and it spearheaded major insights in our understanding of pain. Drs. Melzack and Wall considered the earlier view of hard-wired pain as simplistic and became its major opponents.[17]

Dr. Wall had an interesting view. He considered that the perception of pain (the final step of the process we discussed earlier) is an attempt by the nervous system to achieve dynamic stability—a way of seeking balance. He cites the example of a plane flying a steady course on autopilot. The autopilot receives precisely defined inputs from a multiplicity of sensors and sends simple outputs to the engines and control systems. The whole ensemble is in "stable function," but all the components are in a "dynamic looped interaction." To understand a dynamic model of pain, according to Dr. Wall, we "need to consider the brain and the whole creature beyond the input."

The old concept of separating the mind from the body has been with us since 1664, attributed to Descartes, who famously said "Cogito ergo sum" (I think, therefore I am). In the Cartesian model, pain is a simple response to a harmful stimulus; it will go away when the injury goes away, and if it happens to generate any adverse emotions, these emotions are a simple accompaniment of the stimulus and will also go away when the injury heals.

We know now that the relationship between an injury and pain is not simple and straightforward. Clinical psychologists and clinicians repeatedly have observed tremendous variations between individuals with the same type of injury. These variations cannot be explained by a simple one-to-one relation between the amount of tissue damage or the extent of an injury and the degree or intensity of pain the individual feels. It is only in the last 10 to 15 years that tremendous advances have been made in our understanding of the dynamic mechanisms of pain, beyond the simple concept of definable hard-wired pathways.

These advances became possible when scientists managed to study brain activity without the need to actually open the skull. Different forms of brain imaging, including PET (positron emitting tomography), fMRI (functional magnetic resonance imaging) and others, have revealed that an incredible array of brain areas are activated during the reception of multiple stimuli (hearing, seeing, repeating an activity, thinking about an action or feeling pain). Surprisingly, the perception of pain generates a tremendous degree of activity in brain areas never expected or believed to be associated with pain. Such areas may be involved with attention and orientation, motor function and emotions. At the Toronto Western Hospital, Dr. Karen Davis and her team studied four different brain activation areas in 12 people using hot and cold stimuli as well as touch stimuli. The most remarkable observation was that when the results were pooled together, all four brain areas showed activity, but not one single person among the 12 had the same pattern of activity as any of the others.[18]

Tissue Damage without Pain

It is relatively easy to understand how pain can be associated with actual tissue damage. The damage is done, and it hurts. But what about those cases where there is tissue damage but no pain?

Some people actually are born with an inability to sense pain; this is called congenital insensitivity to pain. It is an extremely rare group of disorders, which can sometimes run in a family. The first well-studied case of this grouping, done a few years after the Second World War, was a Canadian girl who was a student at McGill University.[19] She had never felt pain, even when she had chewed part of her tongue while eating and sustained serious burns kneeling on a radiator to look outside. Similarly, when tested in the laboratory, she did not feel pain when exposed to very hot water, strong electrical shocks or ice-cold water. Obviously her problem was specific to the sensation of pain, as her intelligence and other body functions were intact.

Eventually, this young woman ended up with serious damage in many of her joints and soft tissues, and required several orthopedic surgeries. This damage was the result of her inability to feel pain, as her body could not warn her when she was placing undue demands on her joints, and maybe also the result of the lack of special chemicals within the nerve fibres that maintain the healthy state of body tissues, as I will discuss later. She ultimately died of a massive infection since her damaged tissues allowed uncontrollable growth of bacteria. There were no obvious abnormalities to be seen in her nervous system, which was examined after her death.[20] This is indeed a remarkable case of blockage of the pain signals somewhere between the body and the brain occurring since birth.

Today we know that congenital insensitivity to pain may encompass more than one cause and may or may not be related to structural abnormalities within the nervous system. Such structural abnormalities may affect different fibres within our nerves, which convey impulses between a part of our body and various regions of the nervous system. The nerves look like a rope made up of many strands or "nerve fibres" of different sizes. In most of us, there is a consistent blend of large and small fibres. An example of small fibres are those that convey pain produced by the tip of a needle (the A-delta and C fibres), while large fibres (A-beta fibres) are those that convey the simple touch of a feather on our skin. In some cases of congenital insensitivity to pain, the large fibres in the nerves are very abnormal, in others, the small fibres are decreased in numbers or missing, or the nerve roots that fan out of the peripheral nerves seem to be damaged as they enter the spinal cord. In some of these unfortunate cases, instead of abnormal nerve fibres, there may be abnormalities in certain genes that control chemicals regulating pain signals.

Certain diseases as well can make a person insensitive to pain later in life. Cavities within the spinal cord, which occur in people who have a disorder called syringomyelia, or conditions that affect peripheral nerves as in cases of long-standing diabetes (diabetic neuropathy) or leprosy can be associated with insensitivity to pain. Insensitivity to pain (since birth as in the case of the young woman I discussed earlier, or due to disorders occurring later in life) can lead to damaged joints (called "Charcot's joints" after the physician who first described them) and soft tissues, which in turn can cause infections and require amputations. Previously it was believed that the tissue damage was exclusively due to the lack of the protective effect of pain as a warning signal—a sign telling us to move or change positions. But now we believe that there can be additional causes. Joint and tissue damage can also be due to a lack of "neurotrophic factors" (chemicals released when signals are transmitted between body parts and nerves), the interaction between a defective nervous system and the blood flow to the bones and joints, or a combination of these factors.[21]

However, you don't need a defective nervous system to block pain. Billions of people—perhaps all of us—block pain at one time or another, even if only temporarily. Wounded soldiers hurt in battle or football players injured during the game may truly not feel pain at the time of injury. They will feel it later, but what is it that stops them from experiencing pain when the injury happens? How does the transition from acute to chronic pain occur? What really happens when there is an injury but no pain, or when pain exists after the injury has healed? What about pain that is out of proportion to the injury? I will try to answer these and many other questions in upcoming chapters.

Three

MEN AND WOMEN

Clara came into my office for the first time in January of 1991. She was then 58 years old and was suffering from diffuse pains, which had appeared gradually in her buttocks. Twenty years earlier she had fallen at work and since then she would complain of the odd back pain. However, Clara was never clear whether the buttock pains were related to that old incident, and neither was I. She also said that some years ago she had suffered from a "nervous breakdown."

Clara had immigrated to Canada from Italy at the age of 21. She had two married sons and continued to work as a cashier four hours a day for many years in a local food store. I examined Clara thoroughly and ordered some tests. Except for a little bit of arthritis in her spine I could not find much. I sent her for physiotherapy, which produced minimal improvement. As I kept following Clara over several years, she progressively developed other pains in different body areas. Her sleep was bad, her moods were up and down and she was in constant pain. She would visit me every few months with the same litany of complaints. So far, she has made the rounds of my clinic, and had seen several other consultants in rheumatology, neurology, nephrology, psychiatry and more. Numerous medications had been tried and they all failed or caused her side effects, even when in "baby" doses. Physiotherapy sessions and exercises also failed to help. Her husband had developed heart trouble over the previous three years, and so, in addition to suffering physical pain, Clara felt overburdened. Since her husband's heart problems began, Clara's visits and complaints to me and the other doctors increased considerably. At one point, Clara was diagnosed with fibromyalgia, a disorder that to me and many other physicians (though not all) means diffuse body pains due to heightened sensitivity. Remarkably, the only time that Clara felt better was whenever she would go on vacation back to Italy.

Nicolette was 31 when her doctor sent her to me for "tail bone pain." Six months before I saw her at our pain program she had undergone a rectal surgery for hemorrhoids. Since then she had continuous pain at the tip of her tail bone, called the coccyx, which was worse when she was sitting or walking. Her doctors looked into the possibility of bone fracture, infection or inflammation and questioned whether she had suffered nerve damage during the surgery. However, when I took a careful history I realized that my patient had many long-standing pain problems. Actually, Nicolette had had low back pain since the age of 14 and had seen many doctors for this. She had all kinds of tests and medications, including some powerful painkillers such as morphine, which did not work even at high doses. On top of all this, Nicolette had undergone at least 21 abdominal surgeries, including laparoscopies, laparotomies, appendectomy, gall bladder surgery, total hysterectomy and removal of both her ovaries. All these abdominal surgeries were done for endometriosis and abdominal/pelvic pain but they did not seem to help. Nicolette came accompanied by her husband, who remained present throughout the interview and the physical examination and seemed very caring and attentive. During the examination Nicolette walked slowly and rarely smiled. When I examined the area between her buttock crease, sensation was normal and I failed to find any considerable tenderness except very mild discomfort at the tip of the coccyx. I found no signs whatever of nerve injury. As a matter of fact, there was nothing much to find at the tip of her coccyx, which was the primary reason for her referral. Nicolette did not volunteer any information about previous psychiatric history or depression, something that pain physicians must always ask about. Thank God, the

general population? How long do these ailments last? What is the cost to society? What are the signs and symptoms? All of these epidemiological questions can be applied to chronic pain.

An epidemiologist will approach the issue of chronic pain from different angles. First, he or she will look at the *population* perspective, studying conditions both in the general population and in persons specifically seeking treatment by visiting health care facilities. Second, the researcher will look at the *developmental* perspective; this is when pain is studied across the life cycle, since pain conditions may vary with age or hormones. Finally, an epidemiologist will look at the *ecological* perspective, so we can understand how and when the person's characteristics interact with the environment for a disease to be manifested.

When it comes to pain research, women traditionally have been excluded as research subjects. This was partially because researchers assumed that the results produced by studies of pain in men could be generalized to women too. This has changed. While for many years we pursued equality of the sexes, it is only during the last couple of decades that scientists have agreed to acknowledge and discuss potentially important differences. Dramatic progress in pain research and sweeping changes in cultural attitudes have revolutionized the field of research on sex-related differences in pain responses.[1]

Recent epidemiological reviews show that the prevalence of many pain conditions appears higher in women than men.[2] *Prevalence* is a term used by epidemiologists to indicate the "proportion of persons in the population with a given condition or disease at a particular time." In the laboratory, when men and women are tested specifically for pain, women have lower pain thresholds and can tolerate pain less when compared to men.[3] A summary of recent epidemiological studies across many pain syndromes shows that women have higher rates of general headaches (up to three times more), migraines (up to four times more), temporomandibular disorders (pains associated with the jaw; up to 2.6 times more), "burning mouth syndrome" (up to 2.5 times more), shoulder pain (up to 2.2 times more), knee pain (up to 1.9 times more) and fibromyalgia (up to 6.8 times more).[4] In general, at least up to age 65, women are more likely to experience pain than men, particularly when it comes to pain in multiple body regions. However, some pain syndromes studies show conflicting findings, and one has to be careful how to interpret these results.

For example, the pattern of back pain, one of the most common pain conditions, is not consistent; some studies find higher rates of back pain in women than men but others don't. It may be that other factors, such as the differences between people living in cities versus those living in the country or socio-economic differences, are so powerful that it becomes impossible to identify the exact degree of influence exerted by gender or age.

The relationship between sex and pain is not simple. While several conditions may be more prevalent in women, the prevalence rates vary from disorder to disorder or across the life cycle. But even with all these caveats, the mere fact that research consistently shows that several pain conditions are seen more frequently in women than in men indicates that there might be some distinct common factors specific to females.

A good way of looking at sex-related differences in our perception of pain is to accept and recognize that the experience of pain is the composite sum of complex and dynamic interactions—a mixture of biological, psychological, social and cultural factors. The *biopsychosocial* approach to this and all other aspects of the study of pain is a pivotal concept of understanding in general health and disease.[5] Because it shows how complex the pain experience is, this is a model we will return to frequently.

Pain and Biology

To understand differences between men and women, it is important first of all to define "gender" as opposed to "sex." While these terms are often considered interchangeable, in my discussions I will use the word "sex" to refer to biologically determined aspects of our existence as males and females, and "gender" to refer to social and culturally shaped and modifiable traits such as femininity and masculinity.[6] For example, the way we dress is shaped by the type of society we live in. In the Western world it is socially acceptable for women to wear dresses, skirts or pants. However, a man wearing a skirt in the Western world certainly will raise some eyebrows (unless he lives in Scotland).

There is no question that women differ from men in several ways and in terms of many senses, not just pain. Recent decades have seen two contradictory processes—the development of scientific research looking at the differences between the sexes and the political minimization of such differences.[7] The first systematic attempt to explore sex differences started with Francis Gatton in 1882, at the South Kensington Museum in London, England.[8] Issues arose during the creation of standard IQ tests in the 1950s, to the point where the doctor who developed the most commonly used IQ tests had to admit that ". . . our findings do confirm . . . that men not only behave but 'think' differently than women."[9]

The reality of differences between men and women is overwhelming. Boys outnumber girls four to one in remedial reading classes, stuttering and other speech defects occur almost exclusively in boys and more than six times as many girls than boys can sing in tune.[10] For many decades, these differences were chalked up to "society." However, the popular jokes about women's ability (or to say it better, "inability") to read a map actually do have some scientific basis—men, for example, seem to have better visual-spatial skills. They also seem to perform better in mathematics, have superior hand-eye co-ordination for ball sports and are more capable in seeing patterns and abstract relationships.[11] On the other hand, women are more capable of receiving a wider range of sensory information; they speak earlier in life and more fluently, and hear better than men. They also see better in the dark, are more sensitive to red light and have wider peripheral vision. Women truly see the "bigger picture," as they possess more of the specialized vision receptors called rods and cones in their retinas. Women have an enhanced sense of taste of certain substances and greater sensitivity to sound, particularly in higher frequencies, while their sense of smell is generally better than that of men, a sense that gets enhanced just before ovulation.[12] Women are more sensitive to touch as well.[13] Interestingly, men can recognize faces faster when the pictures are presented to their left visual field (the pictures therefore end up in the right side of the brain) than when the pictures are presented to the other side and are received in their left hemispheres. This doesn't happen to women.[14]

When it comes to pain, women again prove to be more sensitive than men. For example, when women were tested in their breasts and the skin around their nipples, they felt more pain than men. This sensitivity, however, becomes apparent only after puberty.[15] The fluctuation of sensitivity to pain and other sensory stimuli depending on the phase of the menstrual cycle explains the common and long-held preference of aestheticians not to wax a woman's legs if she is at a certain stage prior to her period. While *individual* males and females may share certain responses and perceptions, as a whole, there is no question in the mind of scientists that men and women sense differently the world in general and pain in particular.

The differences can sometimes be readily apparent, but other times they are subtle and complex and multiple factors are responsible for them. Let's start with the obvious differences, our hormones.

The sex (gonadal) hormones in male and female animals as well as in humans are called androgens and estrogens. These gonadal hormones are necessary not only for reproduction; they seem to affect all body regions and neural circuits. Secretion of these hormones in certain periods of life, for example during pregnancy or just after delivery, cause permanent changes in many systems. Gonadal hormones can also modulate the functions of the central nervous system throughout life. Even when we are adults, our brains remain remarkably responsive to the effects of these hormones.

All gonadal hormones (male and female) are derived from cholesterol through a pathway that contains a number of steps. The final step in this pathway produces the female hormone estradiol, which is secreted in large quantities by the ovaries in women who are not pregnant, or the placenta (the sac that contains the embryo) in women who are pregnant. Certain receptors (specialized nerve endings) respond to estradiol; one type is found in many viscera (like the uterus, the testes and the kidneys), while another type of estradiol receptors is found in the brain, the lung and the urinary bladder.

Testosterone (the male gonadal hormone) on the other hand is synthesized in specialized cells in the testes and has only one kind of receptor. These male hormone receptors exist in many structures of the body, including the spinal cord and the brain. Estradiol and testosterone regulate the reading (transcription) of several genes. As well, they fine-tune and modulate certain nervous system actions such as learning and memory. Estrogens affect cognitive function and alter mood and sense of well-being, as women and their partners know well.

Estrogens also have specific effects on the cardiovascular system. This can be seen through the much lower rate of heart conditions in premenopausal women. These effects have been attributed to the action of estrogens on the wall of the blood vessels.[16]

In the nervous system, estrogens seem to exert their actions in many locations, for example, the dorsal root ganglia, the spinal cord, the thalamus and the brain. The fact that there are estrogen receptors in the dorsal root ganglia (which contain the cells of pain fibres like A-delta and C) makes us think that maybe abnormal neuronal activity in these structures also contributes to chronic pain in women. In experiments involving animals, during pregnancy the pain threshold for certain painful events seems to be increased; in other words, the animals feel less pain. This effect seems to take place at the spinal cord, where increased estrogens throughout pregnancy enhance the levels of endogenous opioids, the internal, morphine-like painkilling substances (as we discussed in chapter two).

The brain, as well, seems to develop differently between men and women thanks to the secretion of hormones during the early stages just after conception and throughout life. Up to six or seven weeks after conception, the human embryo is neither male nor female. Around that time, however, it truly "makes up its mind."[17] Our genes will help direct which way the embryo will go (determining whether it will become a girl or a boy). Mammals have 23 pairs of chromosomes, which house together anywhere between 50,000 to 150,000 genes. The last pair of chromosomes determines (partially) the sex of the child. The baby must carry one chromosome per pair from each of the parents. An X chromosome is always given by the mother. The father, however, may give either an X or a Y chromosome. The combination XX in the embryo will create a baby girl, while the combination XY will create a baby boy . . . if hormones intervene when they should. If secreted, the male hormones will be the ones that determine a child's sex. If a female fetus that carries the XX chromosomes is exposed to the male hormones at the crucial time of six weeks after conception, it will be born as a normal-looking male. If a fetus carrying the XY combination is deprived of the crucial male hormones at six weeks, the newborn baby will look exactly like a normal girl. In other words, secretion of the male hormones at this crucial time of development will tell the body to develop male genitalia and not bother developing female genitalia.[18] In male babies an inordinate shower of male hormones is needed not only to shape the external genitalia but to organize the brain in a male pattern. Ample scientific work with rats, birds and monkeys has shown that hormones affect behaviours and that they also affect neural structures (size and shape) and their wiring—

the neural connections.[19] Later in life, male or female hormones in spurts (during adolescence) or through the life cycle will continue to affect behaviours and body functions.

Again, when it comes to pain, the gonadal hormones play an active role in modulating the balance of a number of neurotransmitters in the nervous system, such as norepinephrine and acetylcholine or serotonin. It is important for those trying to understand pain to keep this information in mind, as certain abnormalities in neurotransmitters have been found in some human chronic pain syndromes. As well, the gonadal hormones influence the body's internal painkillers, the endogenous opioid system. In women, these gonadal hormones alter certain pain thresholds or the ability to feel painful stimuli, depending on the stage of the menstrual cycle.[20] Clinical practitioners find that certain human conditions are significantly related to reproductive life events. For example, the menstrual period produces maximal vulnerability to migraine attacks, which females suffer more than males.

So, gonadal hormones are necessary not only for reproduction; in reality, there is no body region or circuit that is not affected by them. Scientists may not know the exact mechanisms by which sex hormones influence pain perception, but to cite a few possibilities, sex hormones may affect metabolism (this has implications for drug use), the immune system, trauma-induced inflammation and the nervous system. However, the profound importance of social and cultural factors as well as psychological factors in pain perception should not be forgotten.

Beyond our hormones, men and women differ in the way they respond to analgesic drugs and in the mobilization of internal painkillers (endogenous analgesia systems). Such differences have been shown to exist in the laboratory with rats and mice, as well as in the clinic. Men and women may react differently to certain types of drugs, sometimes simply by virtue of being human, at other times by virtue of being male or female. It may come as a surprise to some, but it is only during the last decade that the U.S. Food and Drug Administration (FDA) has recognized the need to include women in drug studies and developed new guidelines for pain research. So far, we know surprisingly little about sex-related differences in response to different medications. Only one study has looked at the responses of men and women to the well-known non-steroidal anti-inflammatory drug (NSAID) ibuprofen, which works in similar ways to Aspirin. The findings suggested that women respond less to this drug.[21] Regarding the response to strong pain killers like opioids, several studies show that men require more opioid analgesics to relieve post-operative pain, while in other studies the results are conflicting.[22] Yet when it comes to a certain class of opioid drugs interacting with a specific type of opioid receptors (the κ receptors), women respond better than men. It seems obvious that if differences exist between men and women in their responses to drugs, this will have implications when it comes to the treatment of human painful disorders. Again, from the biological perspective, many of the differences may be influenced by genes, hormones or both. But since biology is intermingled with our psyche and our environment and culture, things get more complex.

Of course, some painful events occur exclusively in females. Any woman who has had a baby can attest to this. Pregnancy and labour are highly stressful and energy-consuming physiological processes. Modulation of pregnancy and labour-related pain is not only desirable but also beneficial to both the mother and the baby. "Antinociceptive" or "anti-pain" effects have been confirmed in pregnant women and in laboratory rats that respond less and less to pain from electrical shocks as pregnancy progresses. This effect peaks just before delivery and seems to be due to increased release of the endogenous opioids as a response to the large amounts of hormones during pregnancy.[23]

Another perhaps more interesting topic specific to females and the act of reproduction relates to analgesia occurring during vaginal stimulation, discussed earlier. Only during the last decade or so have data (from both female rats and women) provided clear evidence that stimulation of the vagina and cervix can produce analgesia . . . not only does "it feel good," it's a painkiller!

Years later, when vaginal stimulation-induced analgesia was confirmed by several laboratories in animals and humans, the researchers started comparing this form of analgesia with stress-induced analgesia generated by stressful stimuli, such as a jolt of electrical current or exposure to cold environment.[24] The scientists concluded that vaginal stimulation-induced analgesia is a form of stress-induced analgesia, provided we accept that stress does not have to be aversive but can be also pleasurable. Heart rate and blood pressure double during orgasm in women, which means that orgasm generates a high level of stress. However, the experience of orgasm is extremely pleasurable. In the same line, skydiving, car racing, intensely physical sports or riding a roller coaster are stressful, but can generate profound excitement. It seems, then, that "bad" stress and "good" stress are both associated with release of the body's own pain killers.

Interestingly, when it comes to vaginal and cervical stimulation, we can feel either pleasure, pain or analgesia or all of these at once. The interaction of the mind and the body can produce startlingly different results even if the physical stimulus is, objectively speaking, not all that different—lovemaking may produce intense pleasure, while a rape will cause pain, as it is accompanied by extremely negative emotions.

It isn't prurience that leads researchers to gather information about pain and pleasure responses during sex. The information may help develop sex-specific strategies for pain treatments.

Men, Women and Sociocultural Influences

What about cultural differences? Gender, ethnicity and culture are parts of our personal identity. While being a man or woman is a matter of biology, our social setting affects us greatly too. Two different males with the exact same ethnic background may respond entirely differently to pain as adults. Their biological and genetic characteristics are important, but their responsiveness to pain depends also on whether they grew up in Stockholm or Rome, on the behavioural expectations within their families and cultures and also on the way people of their background are viewed by people of other cultures where they live.[25]

Again, a person's sex is not the same as his or her gender. Gender encompasses something larger—it includes social and cultural traits that can be learned and shaped, such as femininity and masculinity. The experts don't all agree on how we acquire our gender. Some psychologists propose that we develop our sense of male or female gender through learning processes such as modelling, imitation, reinforcement and punishment. Others insist that we acquire our female or male gender by conforming to cultural stereotypes for these traits.[26] Gender traits may develop early in life or later on, depending on the circumstances.

When it comes to pain and the way we react to it, there is no question that gender role expectations and social role modelling of reactions to pain may interact early in life. Research has shown that young boys "tough it out" to conform to perceived expectations that boys are more able than girls to take pain.

Men and women not only feel pain but tell others about pain differently. In one study, when subjects were asked to rate imagined pain in several body parts, men seemed to react to pain with embarrassment and said they would be reluctant to complain about it, while women became anxious and admitted that they were highly likely to tell others about their pain.[27]

Gender stereotyping plays an important role in shaping our own ideas about our masculinity or femininity and also in shaping our reaction to the opposite sex. Men reported less pain during a test exposing them to a painfully cold stimulus if the experimenter was a good-looking 28-year-old woman dressed provocatively. No such effects were observed if the experimenter was a man or if the woman was dressed in a neutral or unattractive way.[28] In another experiment, researchers tested men who scored high on a particular "masculinity scale."[29] These men actually saw themselves as "very manly" and were compared with men who scored low in the same scale. The researchers presented the experimental subjects with a particularly painful experiment. When the task was presented as a "masculine achievement task," those who scored high on the masculinity scale had higher increases in their blood pressure. The researchers concluded that the masculine challenge was particularly stressful and threatening for those men who were conforming to the more stereotypically masculine images. Similarly, in other experiments women showed stronger reactions in the "feminine challenge" condition. These experiments indicate to me that when our masculinity or femininity is challenged, we are more stressed out and anxious.

I have certainly seen gender stereotyping, and how it shapes pain behaviour, throughout my whole life, both as a Greek woman and as a professional. My father was born in Southern Peloponnesus in Greece, in a region called Mani, which is for Greece what Sicily is for Italy—a region with a tight, self-enclosed moral universe. My Dad told me a story that for me epitomizes the local culture. When a man's wife was giving birth he would proudly announce to the other village people (usually males sitting in the local *kafenion*) that he "got a child" if the baby was a boy, while a female infant would be announced just as "a girl."

My mother used to tell me that older women arranging marriages would tell the young future brides that "a man need not be beautiful, just being a man is enough." In my Greek culture we understood that "men do not cry," "men are strong," "they do not display emotions," "they take it like a man" and, let's not forget this one, "they are non-stop sex machines." Even through my high school years, I remember that my girlfriends and I would question the sexual orientation of any soft-spoken gentleman or anyone who would display his feelings or complain about things (as if gentleness and manhood were incompatible).

Today, I know better how to tell myths from truth, and my understanding of stereotyped gender roles has evolved. When I was an intern in my early 20s in Athens, it was not unusual to see tall, "manly" men coming to my hospital for blood testing. Some would nearly faint at the sight of the needle and get drenched in sweat as it punctured their veins. Perhaps these men were unable to abide by what was stereotypically expected of them, or maybe deep in their hearts they didn't really believe that "men never cry." But a man does not have to be a Greek to react this way. A colleague in my hospital, urologist Dr. Sidney Radomsky, tells me that many more men than women grow faint on his examining table during cystoscopy, when he passes a thin tube into the male or female urethra to see the urinary bladder. Maybe we women are so used to submitting ourselves to the "legs up position" on the gynecologist's table that this does not bother us as much. On the other hand, the clichés seem true—the epicentre of manliness seems to be exclusively located in this small area between a man's two pelvic bones. It seems to me that this fixed idea of what makes a man a "real man" recognizes no cultures or borders.

The stereotyped gender role is exemplified for me by a case I encountered early in my career. Gus was a tall, muscular Greek in his mid-40s who had been in Canada at least 20 years when he came to see me. His English was rather poor, but this did not bother me, as we talked in Greek. Gus had a very bad knee and a bad stomach. He could not take aspirin-like drugs of any sort and he had no time for physiotherapy. He hated needles, so he rejected my offer for a knee injection. Finally, I said that the only thing I could do for him was to give him suppositories containing the drug. I hoped that bypassing the stomach route would result in less stomach burning and irritation. Gus did not know what a suppository was. I proceeded to explain.

Gus's face turned red like a tomato: "You . . .," he gasped. "How do you dare! Nobody sticks a finger or anything else in my ass!" Gus would rather take the pain in his knee than submit himself to what he perceived as a humiliation. From that day on, I became more cautious when it came to treatments or tests of any sort that may be considered a threat to a man's self-image. Yet I have not encountered similar problems with women, maybe because they feel comfortable with me being a woman too.

Feelings, Thoughts and Gender Differences

Pain is subjective. The gate control theory of pain, discussed earlier, accepts that our experience of pain is influenced by biological, psychological and psychosocial experiences. But when it comes to the way we face problems, men and women's thought processes are different.

In general, men and women cope with stress differently. Men tend to concentrate more on problem-solving strategies while women focus more on the interpersonal and emotional aspects of the situation. Pain certainly can be defined as a stressor. A few studies indicate that when it comes to pain, women rely more on social and emotional support than men.[30] When men and women appraise a painful situation, more men than women feel that they are "in control" of their pain and report low levels of pain and less "catastrophizing"— thinking of an experience as a catastrophe. Catastrophizing has been recognized as an important contributor to pain perception and affects the outcome of pain treatments.[31] Catastrophizing is characterized by feelings of lack of control, excessive worry about the future and a sense that life is overwhelming. It bears an important relationship to chronic pain. When individuals are tested in a laboratory, catastrophizing and culture seem to play a role in their reactions to pain.

Research has shown that pain and unpleasant emotions go hand in hand. This may seem obvious if you have ever smashed your thumb with a hammer, but its significance goes beyond the obvious. Negative emotions like anger, fear and depression may increase the sensitivity of our bodies and result in more pain. On the other hand, pain by itself may lead to negative emotions. Women tend to report more psychological distress than men in general and this may contribute to the sex differences in the experience of pain.[32] One researcher noted that increased awareness of one's body and depression was found in women but not men with low back pain. She suggested that maybe it is more "socially acceptable for women to admit to distress than men . . . ."[33] Other studies as well have found differences between headache sufferers, with women reporting greater psychological distress. Maybe women's multiple roles—house-keeping, parenting and working outside the home—are overwhelming and contribute to their increased perception of pain.[34]

Men and women are also different in how they utilize health care services. Women use these services more for all types of diseases. This explains the much greater numbers of women than men that attend my clinic and other pain clinics. On the other hand, women are 3.6 times more likely to listen to the advice of the doctor when the doctor prescribes a restriction of activities. Overall, health care utilization is influenced significantly by different health beliefs, concerns and perception of symptoms between the two sexes. Furthermore, the social welfare or disability system is used differently by men and women. In a study of injured workers, researchers showed that men returned to work sooner than women but were more likely to become disabled again. Women took longer to return to work but managed to stay in the work-force once they started working. Perhaps women's additional duties at home prolonged their time off work, but once back at work, they were there to stay.

Men and women should remember that we differ in our behaviours; communication style; the way we dress, work or play; our coping with stress in general and pain in particular; our ways of expressing sorrow and sadness, anxiety, anger or happiness. However, we should also remember that our differences (as well as our similarities) are fundamentally influenced by both our social learning and social milieu, as well as by our biology.

Four

BLOCKING PAIN

At the start of my career, I was asked to see a young woman with chronic pain in both knees. She had gone through the rounds of many physicians over the decade. Little had been found wrong with her despite many tests. Jane walked into my office with two canes. She was 33 years old, bright, good looking and slim, a part-time university student in philosophy and a single mother of a five-year-old boy. I took a careful history and then thoroughly examined her knees. Except for a bit of tenderness I was unable to find much to explain her unrelenting, incapacitating pain—no cracking sounds, no water in her knees, no changes in colour, temperature or sensation. With such an unimpressive examination, I spoke frankly to Jane and said that I would repeat a couple of tests, but I warned her that I did not really expect to find anything remarkably wrong. I also told her that I probably was not going to come up with a miraculous treatment either. In those days of the early 1980s, when there was less strain on the health care system, I could order all kinds of tests and get them done within days. So I asked Jane to have some knee X-rays and a bone scan. For a bone scan, we inject the patient with a special tracer (a substance marked by a radioactive material so it can be traced on a film). This material has a special tendency to concentrate in the bones. Fractures, inflammation, degenerative changes and all other kinds of physical problems will easily show up with such a test.

Jane came back to see me 10 days later. By then I had received the test results. As I had predicted, I could see nothing wrong with her knees. But . . . to my surprise, the bone scan showed a "hot spot" in her left rib cage, indicating a recent rib fracture. Jane had never mentioned anything about chest pain in our first encounter.

"So," I asked her, "did you hurt your chest lately?"

"Oh yes," she replied candidly. "A couple of days before my appointment with you, I fell off the stairs and cracked a rib. My family doctor told me that's what it is."

"For goodness' sake," I exclaimed, "we spent one and a half hours talking about your knee pain and you never said a word about this other 'fresh' pain! Doesn't it hurt?"

"Of course," she stressed. "It stings. But it's easy for me to control it."

"How?"

"My doctor has explained the anatomy of the ribs to me. When I close my eyes I imagine the two parts of the broken rib coming closer and closer to each other. Once they touch each other, the pain goes."

"For the life of me," I blurted in frustration. "Here you have this 'physical' pain which I know hurts a lot, and you can block it to the point you did not even bother to discuss it with me. On the other hand, you suffer 10 years from this 'ghost' pain for which there is nothing much of a physical nature, and you are incapacitated. Can't you use the same method of imagery to control the knee pains too?"

"No," she shouted. "I have a big problem. I do not understand the anatomy of the knees. I haven't been told anything about any process that might disturb this anatomy, so I can't 'imagine' anything to block the pain!"

Jane's ability to "block" pain produced by actual physical damage, using a technique called imagery, came as a major surprise to me. I was fresh, just a couple of years out of my residency training, suffering from the complex most young doctors experience: a blend of arrogance, ignorance and the confidence that we know a lot (at least, "what the books say") and that our "medical model of disease" has equipped us well to understand the vast majority of human ailments. Nothing was further from the truth. Over the many years that went by after I saw Jane, my patients have continued to challenge me with many symptoms and signs that did not fit what I was taught and were not written "in the books." In case after case, I would discover how intense and bizarre the influence of the "mind" is on all aspects of pain perception and expression.

As we try to understand how Jane and others block pain, we must distinguish the primary sensory experience that stems from a noxious stimulus (what scientists really mean when they talk about "pain") and our reaction to this sensory experience (lay people call this pain too, but it really means our "suffering"). Pain and suffering are intimately intertwined, but they can also be distinguished as separate components of our pain experience. The distinction has really come to light during studies of people who had frontal lobotomies for the control of intractable pain. These patients were still able to localize the pain—they could perceive the sensory experience—but they did not react to it. Because they had lost the unpleasantness of the experience they were not suffering any more.

Pain is an integral part of every living organism. Pain is a natural consequence of childbirth. Pain can be the product of diseases, injuries or even the result of their treatments; this is why people with chronic pain come to see doctors like me. Pain can be inflicted by humans on fellow humans as well, in the form of torture or punishment. Some of my patients who come to Canada from war- and terror-torn countries have intense physical and emotional scars and long-lasting pain and suffering. Pain under most circumstances is not welcome. To combat it, people all over the world have used methods that vary from the very primitive to the most sophisticated and technologically advanced. Alcohol, for example, has been known since antiquity to be an excellent pain reliever, as it dulls all senses. This is why when we see a drunk at a party we might remark that he or she is "feeling no pain."

I certainly know the painkilling properties of alcohol from first-hand observation. In my early years of training, I spent a few months in an orthopedic hospital emergency in a suburb of Athens. I still remember vividly the pervasive licorice-sweet smell of ouzo (a famous Greek liqueur that turns opaque when mixed with water) or the sharp smell of retsina (Greek resin-flavoured wine) filling the crowded emergency room, as a drunk was brought by ambulance with a shoulder out of its socket. He would hardly complain of pain as the doctor, with a gentle but steady pull, would put back the shoulder. Certainly if the man were sober he would need to breathe some form of quick-acting anaesthetic before he would allow anyone to manipulate this shoulder. Alcohol is not the only remedy used as a painkiller, of course. In Malaysia and areas of the Far East, tribal doctors use "charm needles." These little needles are inserted deep under the skin of the face, chest, abdomen and other areas to treat numerous conditions ranging from infections to pain.[1] Unlike acupuncture, in which needles are inserted for a short time, these needles are left under the skin indefinitely—often forever. It may not seem immediately obvious, but it's not that great a leap from this to sophisticated Western methods of pain control, such as the use of electrical stimulators with wires that are implanted into nerves, the spinal cord or the brain.

Rituals and Pain

All along we have talked about efforts to harness pain. But in certain parts of the world, extraordinary trauma to the human flesh is sometimes inflicted on people without any indication of discomfort. In India, the Middle and Far East, Africa, in certain countries of Europe and among North American First Nations, enduring pain is sometimes considered a proof of divinity, a demonstration of faith or preparedness to "become an adult" during initiations or other rituals. Despite procedures that can be extremely gruesome, there is little damage to the body. Such rituals are foreign to the traditional Western culture in which I live and practise medicine, and they have challenged, amazed and provoked scientists for many years. Jane's story was a real jolt for me and it slowly opened the door toward my understanding of the ways the human spirit can block pain.

In the 1980s I used to watch the late shows on TV. Occasionally my attention would be caught by a very tall young man with prominent horse-like jaws speaking passionately about the power of mind over the body (I later learned his name was Anthony Robbins). He used to brag about his methods of empowering thousands of followers who had commissioned his services for considerable fees. On late-night TV, he would demonstrate mind over matter by showing devoted followers walking over fire pits. It was all very unusual in a Western context (outside the circus, at least), but fire-walking is not a new phenomenon.

Fire-walking is practised throughout the world and in many cultures. The first written report we have comes from 1200 BC; it describes two priests in India who would walk on fire to show who was the better Brahmin.[2] Around the time of Christ, the Greek geographer Strabo described priestesses walking over glowing coals.[3] In another example, from Persia, the contemporary view was that the priestesses were not burnt because they were inspired by the gods. In the Bible, Isaiah makes reference to faith in the power of God: "When thou walkest through fire, thou shalt not be burned" (Isa. 43:2).

Fire-walking is quite popular on the island of Fiji. In 1973, the Fijians, realizing the commercial possibilities of their fire-walking skills, took their "show on the road" in 37 appearances at hotels in Canada and Hawaii.[4] Today, fire-walking is still practised in the Churches of God and Free Pentecostal Holiness in North America, in Siberia, parts of Europe (including my native Greece), Africa, India, Sri Lanka, Japan and Polynesia.

But what is the explanation behind this phenomenon? Is it based on science or trickery, or does one need a certain state of mind that protects from physical injuries and obliterates pain? Fire-walking was reported in a scientific journal for the first time in 1935 by a British scientist.[5] His report described Kuda Bux, a Kashmiri Indian, whom the scientist studied during two demonstrations of fire-walking. On each occasion Kuda Bux took four steps in less than four seconds to cross a trough of hot coals, and did not get burned. Another scientist who attended those demonstrations contended that fire-walking was really "a gymnastic feat," as his calculations showed that the contact period of each foot with the hot coals was only half a second and this time was short enough to not allow blisters to develop.[6] In 1936, another adventurous scientist walked across flaming red-hot embers in plain socks without "singing, scorching and blistering."[7] He stressed that his feet were protected from getting burnt because of the presence of ash, their cold temperature as a result of his bathing before the ritual, and the nature of stones used. In a series of experiments in 1971, Dr. Carlo Fonseca, professor of physiology at Colombo University in Sri Lanka, found that the length of contact between the hot coals and the feet of those who were not burnt was less than 0.6 seconds.[8] He did not believe that "altered state of mind" or rituals beforehand were needed to achieve "protection from burns." He also stressed, as others had done before, that the state of the feet was another critical factor. Fonseca's science was not well received by the fire-walking devotees in Sri Lanka, who believe that fire-walking is a supernatural phenomenon and that the gods protect the fire-walkers.[9] The devotees of Skanda, the god of Kataragama in Sri Lanka, view fire-walking as "both an act and a test of faith."[10] Sangayama, the president of the fire-walkers and Kataragama devotees, challenged Professor Fonseca in a furious confrontation in public: "What would you say if one could walk over the coals for over a minute without getting burnt?"[11] Fonseca replied that if one could keep one's feet in continuous contact with glowing cinders of 315 to 425°C (600 to 800°F) for more than a minute without sustaining burns, then he was prepared to renounce his science. So far, the validity of Fonseca's concepts has not been challenged.

Still, scientists have persevered in attempting to solve the mystery. A German psychiatrist from Tubingen, Dr. Wolfgang Larbig, together with colleagues, visited Langadas, a small village in Northern Greece. They also studied fire-walkers in Germany between 1978 and 1980. The researchers placed wires in different areas of the skulls of fire-walkers in order to record brain waves, so that they could monitor electroencephalographic recordings (EEGs) over closed-circuit television. Our brains emit different frequencies of waves during activities or sleep. Alpha waves are fairly fast waves occurring at 8 to 13 cycles every second: they are emitted during our regular, conscious activities. Theta waves are slower brain waves at 4 to 7 cycles per second and are normally seen during light sleep or stages of "creative thinking," when we somehow detach ourselves from reality and become absorbed in our thoughts. Larbig's EEG recordings showed that beginner fire-walkers were slipping into theta wave activity, but the more experienced fire-walkers were not.[12] These scientific experiments indicated that while an altered state of mind may be associated with the act of fire-walking, it is not a necessary prerequisite, as not all fire-walkers managed to change their brain waves.

Fire-walking has found commercial applications in the Western world. Numerous fire-walking strolls have been staged by individuals who claim, like the man I used to watch on TV, that the mind can control pain and bodily responses and people can be introduced to powers they never knew they could possess.[13] While this is true, fire-walking by itself is far from being a simple "mind over matter" issue. In 1985, an American hypnotherapist, Hugh Bromiley, indeed took his "coal stroll" to London and invited the public to participate. This particular demonstration was reported in the local press.[14] Those who took part in the walk paid £50 each for the session, which was also attended by the public, the media and some scientists. Each man or woman was asked to write down "all his/her fears." The handwritten notes then were burnt in the flames with a ritualistic fanfare before the walk began. In the meantime, in preparation for the walk, participants stood barefoot in a cold muddy patch in front of the glowing coals, repeatedly chanting a mantra: "cool-wet-grass." Then they walked fast through a 3.7-metre (12-foot) path of burning coals. Almost all walked relatively unscathed, except for a woman who fell into a deep trance and walked more slowly than the rest of the group. This woman suddenly jumped out of the burning path, and . . . guess what? She was burned. While she attributed her burns to "distracted attention," so "her state of mind was no longer protecting her," skeptical observers felt that the opposite had occurred. Her altered state of mind made her walk slowly, giving enough contact time between her feet and the burning coals for her feet to burn. Then her pain jolted her out of her "state of mind" and into safety. Indeed, the renowned pain scientist Professor Patrick Wall and other scientist-observers made similar measurements to those of Carlo Fonseca in Sri Lanka in 1971, and showed again that the brevity of contact with the coals was the protective factor behind a successful fire-walk. The researchers again stressed the importance of the condition of the feet before the walk in contributing to protection from burns.[15] The principle of physics behind walking on hot embers was shown to me in a simple way many years ago, when I was describing to my staff my fascination with fire-walking and the true explanations behind it. My friend and assistant Anna, who was born and raised in Guyana, heard me and said in a matter-of-fact tone: "Yeah, I've done it as a kid and never got burnt. And you know what? I was in no special state of mind. You just have to get your feet dry and walk very fast, man, just very fast!"

But does the mind play any role in fire-walking? Can the mind, if harnessed, exert such amazing powers over the body? Most of those who participate in these walks feel immensely exhilarated by their achievement of overcoming their fears, both of fire-walking and, in their minds, many other personal fears. Some even go into an "altered state of mind," as the EEG recordings of some fire-walkers indicate. For many, the way they feel is a far-reaching experience, and indeed the highlight of such walks. Discovering their inner strength is their true bonus. It is truly an act that needs motivation, courage and willpower. So far so good . . . as long as they observe the principles of physics.

While scientists now know that fire-walking does not necessitate a special state of mind, other phenomena do command powers of the mind unknown to the untrained. I will never forget my fascination and amazement as a youngster in Athens when my father took my sister and me to see a famous Indian fakir who was putting on a show. I was about 10 years old. The fakir was a skinny, sunburned man of undetermined age (anywhere between 40 and 60, I would say) who wore only a wrap around his slim waist. I could not get over him: he sat comfortably on a mattress of nails for at least an hour while performing some eye-popping rituals. He could stick long needles in his cheeks or daggers in his arms with no blood coming out! He always stared ahead as if he were detached from the surroundings, and he did not seem to feel or express any pain (while I had goosebumps just watching him). Many years later, as a clinician and a scientist confronted with the emerging awareness that the mind was a power to reckon with, these memories came back to me and prompted me to try to understand them.

A German psychiatrist, fascinated by the amazing things that fakirs do, investigated a 48-year-old Mongolian man who was doing things similar to those performed by the fakir I had witnessed as a child back home in Athens.[16] He could stick daggers in his neck, pierce his tongue with a sword and prick his arms with long needles without any indication of pain or damage to his flesh. How did this man manage to do such things that defy the way normal individuals feel pain and react to it? The story behind his extraordinary abilities is a fascinating case of self-actualization taken beyond conventional limits. As a child this fakir had suffered from a painful disease and he discovered that if he fixed his gaze to a point far away, he could block his pain. Then, while blocking his pain by staring fixedly ahead, he experimented by piercing his arms with his mother's knitting needles. He perfected his skills and developed a set pattern for his performance. First, he would spend several hours in deep meditation before his show. Then he would perform his act without evidence of pain or flesh damage. The scientists recorded the fakir's behaviour step by step throughout the show and took blood from the veins in his arm and cerebrospinal fluid from his spine through a "spinal tap" (which is performed by inserting a needle at the back of the spine, on the surface of the spinal cord). They also recorded the fakir's brain waves with an EEG. Throughout the half-hour performance, the fakir would stare ahead to some fixed imaginary point and he would not blink for up to five minutes. Normally we flicker our eyes several times every minute. He actually looked as if he were "somewhere else" in space and time, not aware of his surroundings. However, when his act was done, he would return quickly to a normal state of consciousness. Blood testing showed that at the end of the act the fakir's adrenaline levels were high (similar to the adrenaline "rush" thrill-seekers experience), but his endogenous opioids (the body's own painkillers) were not affected. How did he not seem to feel or express pain during his show, when daggers and needles were inserted into his flesh? If he was not fending off pain protected by his own painkillers, what other mechanisms did he use to block pain? The answer probably lies in the man's "altered state of mind" during his act. EEG recordings showed that he was switching his brain waves from alpha rhythm to slower theta waves. Ironically, while the fakir did not feel a hint of pain during his act, he complained bitterly when the staff pricked his arm to take blood for testing after his show, when he was back to a "normal" state of mind.

One open question that science has so far failed to answer relates to the obvious lack of substantial injury to the flesh during the fakir performances. If you and I had a knife stuck into our flesh, we would bleed profusely. Why do these fakirs not bleed much or even at all? Why doesn't their flesh get damaged? These same questions were asked and debated by scientists when they tried to understand another remarkable ritual, hook-hanging.

Hook-hanging is practised primarily by selected Kataragama devotees in Sri Lanka and India as an act of penance and religiosity. Some of the earlier accounts come from southern India and some of the rituals have been observed by scientists.

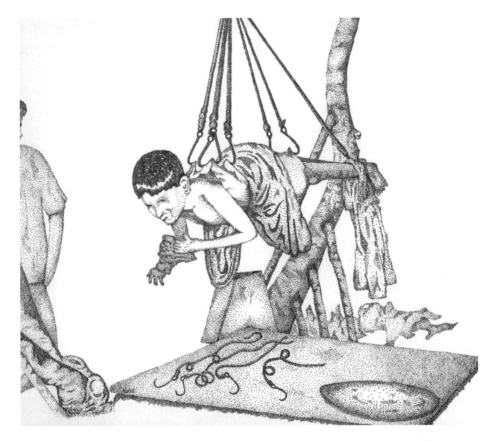

Training for hook-hanging, a ritual practised in Sri Lanka and India, begins in childhood. Practitioners stare at a fixed point and seem to develop a state of mind that allows them to not experience pain during the performance.

Copyright © Norm R. Gagnon. Used with permission.

Dr. Doreen Browne, an anaesthetist from London, England, described what she observed in Sri Lanka in 1983. She noted how the devotees have their flesh pierced by several hooks and are hung and swung from scaffolds over the cheering crowds as they bless the children and the crops. During the whole performance the "hangees" would stare at some fixed point (as the fakir I saw in my childhood did). At no time did any of them seem to experience pain during the gruesome insertion of the hooks, the swinging itself or the removal of the hooks. To the contrary, they seemed to be in a "state of exaltation."[17]

Guananath Obeyesekere, professor of anthropology at the University of California, San Diego, also described in vivid detail the fascinating performance of the ritual he witnessed repeatedly.[18] He confirms again that there is no bleeding when the hooks penetrate the flesh, and the devotee remains in a trance during the performance. One hook-hanger told the scientist that when the hooks pierce his body, "he feels cold as if he [were] in a refrigerator chamber, but no pain." Obeyesekere observed that such rituals seemed to be characteristic of an "arena culture," as they are confined to special times and worship places and are always performed in public. Dr. Browne, the British anaesthetist, quoted her personal communication with an anthropologist in Sri Lanka who told her that the devotees begin "training" in childhood and progress from simple procedures like flesh piercing to hook-hanging.[19] They seem to gradually develop a state of mind unusual for the average person. Hook-hanging has now become part of a modern subculture known as "body mod" (body modification). Displays of people hanging off hooks are shown on "reality" TV shows such as *Ripley's Believe It or Not*. It would be worthwhile to submit these modern hook-hangers to scientific studies of brain waves and body neurochemicals to figure out how they fend off pain.

What fakir phenomena and procedures like hook-hanging have in common is the obvious lack of pain and the lack of tissue damage. The lack of pain may not be that hard to explain. The German psychiatrist Dr. Larbig, fascinated with fakirs, yogis, fire-walkers and hook-hangers, studied some of the hook-hangers in his laboratory. He described to Dr. Browne that EEG studies demonstrated theta wave activity present throughout the insertion of the hooks, the duration of swinging and the hook removal process.[20] So the altered state of mind in fakirs and hook-hangers is one good scientific explanation (but maybe not the only one) for the lack of pain experience. But given the gruesome details of the procedures, how does one explain the lack of gushing wounds? In a 1973 paper, Professor Fonseca hypothesized that the skin does not rip if the body weight is symmetrically distributed between 8 to 12 hooks. He also suggested that closing of the local microcirculation at the points of hook (a process called vasoconstriction) may result from the local release of substances acting on the local blood vessels, even though he could not tell how.[21]

Is Fonseca's hypothesis true? I believe the explanations are much more complex than simple "even weight distribution." I am a firm believer that almost everything we do or feel has a scientific explanation . . . including miracles. In numerous instances, our thoughts and emotions, our convictions and beliefs and our ability to harness them or change them affect the way our nervous system operates, can open up and close blood vessels causing or stopping bleeding, mobilize blood cells and repair forces within the tissues and can even account for stopping our heart and breathing in the absence of any physical cause.

Endorphins and Altered States of Consciousness

One way of blocking pain is the release of the body's own painkillers (endogenous opioids). As I have discussed earlier, a special pain suppression network runs from the midbrain to the medulla and then to the spinal cord. This analgesia network is activated both by electrical stimulation and by morphine and other opioids, including the body's own painkillers. Is this endorphin-mediated pathway involved at all in rituals like the ones we discussed? We know today that vigorous physical exercise showers the body with endorphins.[22] Long-distance runners suppress pain during the "runner's high" and at the same time their levels of endorphins are much increased.[23] Although studies have not been done in tribal cultures that practise customs like hook-hanging, some scientists feel that endorphins may indeed play a substantial role, at least in ecstatic-type rituals that involve violent dance moves, a form of vigorous exercise. For example, during such ecstatic dancing, the Hamadsha, a Moroccan tribe, hyperventilate and slash their heads with knives.[24] But they are not aware of their injuries, nor do they feel pain.

Another way of blocking pain is to change the state of mind, for example with the appearance of theta waves as we saw in fakirs and hook-hangers. Studies of yogis practising transcendental meditation (samadhi) do show altered states of mind. Under normal conditions of alertness our brain operates through fairly fast alpha waves, but a brisk light, a thundering noise or an electrical jolt will disrupt the alpha rhythm. In a meditating yogi, the alpha rhythm cannot be interrupted and remains steady, no matter what happens externally or internally in the yogi's body. So far, studies have indeed confirmed that during samadhi the yogis do not feel anything happening to their body (such as a pinch or immersing their hands in ice-cold water) or around them (strong noises or lights).[25] In other experiments, yogis in deep transcendental meditation may even change their brain waves from alpha to theta. To be perceived as noxious, a stimulus must first pass by the reticular formation before it arrives at the conscious brain. During deep meditation, the yogis seem to dissociate their conscious brain from the reticular formation by blocking the communication between these two levels.

Another way of altering our state of mind is to switch our attentional focus. Scientists only recently learned that paying attention to a stimulus is a major event for the body that precedes the awareness of all sensations. In general, before a stimulus like a glittering light, a sound or a smell comes to the level of awareness, the brain as a whole goes through several steps in an orderly fashion: vigilance, alerting, orientation and attention. At all times, the brain must scan the entire sensory input in order to tell how important a stimulus is. Even before the performance of a motor movement such as reaching for a glass of water, certain brain areas seem to be activated a few milliseconds before the execution of a movement. We know very little, however, about the sequence of mechanisms that trigger our attention.

The technique of "distraction" that produces an attentional shift is well known from ancient times. Pain can be blocked when attention is captured by another event that occurs aside from the reason for hurting. This capacity has been shown in studies involving both animals and humans. A fight, an intense sound, a blinding light, a stimulus in a body part remote from the site of injury, or even startling news, such as discovering you have won the lottery, can produce such a shift. When attention is locked into an event that the brain considers higher on its "priority list," the bizarre and paradoxical event of "injury without pain" can occur.

The most remarkable proof that the "mind reigns supreme" comes from experiences with people who are under hypnosis. To observe the calm face of a patient who undergoes a painful procedure without anaesthesia is an unbelievable experience. Hypnosis was first introduced by Franz Mesmer, an eighteenth-century physician from Austria who is considered to be the father of hypnosis (or mesmerism, as it was originally called). Mesmer claimed that he was able to maintain a harmonious balance in the "universal invisible fluid in the human body" by the use of magnetic rods. Later on, James Braid renamed the process hypnosis, pushing the idea of the power of suggestion. Hypnotic exhibitions invaded the Parisian salons, until a royal commission disputed Mesmer's statements and mesmerism fell into disrepute. Mesmerism then became a subject for jokes, as in Mozart's opera *Don Giovanni*. The predominant image of a hypnotist evolved into that of a man with dark moustache, black eyes and a shiny suit on a stage, who would compel the audience to perform silly and embarrassing acts, as if they had no minds of their own and no choice but to obey his commands.

Dr. Patrick Wall compared the hostility and ridicule directed at Mesmer and mesmerism to "throwing the baby out with the tub water."[26] Wall conceded that while "Mesmer may have been an exhibitionist mountebank charlatan quack, . . . he was clearly an astute observer." By the nineteenth century some famous French doctors such as Ambroise Liebault and Jean Martin Charcot had begun to use hypnosis again. Believing that hypnosis was some form of "induced madness," they used it on patients with "hysterical" paralysis or anaesthesia. While hypnosis was by that time used during some surgeries, its course as an acceptable method of pain control remained quite turbulent. For example, a patient who woke up halfway through a surgery performed under hypnosis sued the University College Hospital in London. It is not surprising then that a well-known surgeon who in 1846 completed the first surgery in England under the influence of ether (the first general anaesthetic, discovered in the United States), remarked: "Gentlemen, the Yankee trick beats the French one." Nevertheless, though still burdened by misunderstanding and mystique, hypnosis gradually emerged as a specific weapon against pain and other afflictions. It took time. Hypnoanaesthesia had been described in a classic monograph by a British surgeon in India in 1846. However, hypnosis as an acceptable method of pain control was not endorsed by the American Medical Association until 1958.

But what does hypnosis do, exactly? The first scientific report of bodily changes observed under hypnotic suggestion appeared in 1917 in one of the top medical journals in the world, *The Lancet*. It was written by Arthur Hadfield, a respected navy doctor, who studied a sailor in England.[27] His subject had suffered shell shock and was treated with hypnotherapy. One day during the session, the doctor jokingly suggested that he was going to touch the man's arm with a hot iron and that this was going to hurt a lot. Instead, he touched him with his bare finger. Under hypnosis, the man withdrew from the doctor's finger as if he were suffering serious pain. By the time he woke up he had forgotten all about his pain. However, an hour later, the sailor walked back into the doctor's office complaining bitterly of pain and showing a big blister full of fluid, surrounded by a ring of redness indicating inflammation. The experiment was repeated several times under very strict conditions of observation, with the arm bandaged and the sailor always watched by observers. Each time, a blister formed wherever Dr. Hadfield's finger had touched the man's arm, as long as the doctor was also suggesting that the blister was painful. *The Lancet* published a photograph of the man's arm showing several blisters that had formed under hypnotic suggestion. Traditional English-speaking scientists ignored this very important paper, which was the first to prove that the power of suggestion can produce specific changes in the body. Similar observations of such phenomena were published in German journals, but the knowledge did not spread to English-speaking countries.

Nearly 30 years later, in 1946, Dr. Robert Moody, a psychiatrist at the Woodside Hospital in London, England, published another scientific paper in *The Lancet*.[28] He reported several patients who years before had experienced the combination of a physical and a serious emotional trauma, such as being tied up and beaten, buried by a bomb blast, hit by a falling beam or immersed for a long time in ice-cold water. The events were so traumatic emotionally that they had been somehow isolated from normal consciousness. Under the influence of hypnosis these patients relived their dreadful experiences and under the eyes of the startled doctor they developed rope marks, bruises, swelling and bleeding, similar to their original injuries many years ago, all accompanied by severe pain for several hours. Moody wrote that "neural pathways undoubtedly exist by which psychic contents may be projected on to the body in a highly specific manner." He also felt that when this traumatic experience finds its way into consciousness, "the original trauma is transferred from the memory and recreated in the body." Again, photographs of these patients confirmed the presence of rope burns or marks during the reliving of the experience many years later.

Few such important observations have found their way into scientific journals and remain primarily in the realm of anecdotes, word of mouth and popular publications. Encounters such as those described by Hadfield and Moody were recounted in a fascinating series of books published by Time-Life Books.[29] Disturbed individuals with profoundly traumatic emotional experiences have been observed to bleed painlessly under conditions of emotional turmoil. The case of "stigmata" appearing in the hands and feet of religious individuals who participate in crucifixion-like ceremonies were critically reviewed by a number of doctors and psychologists in the 1920s. Those scientists started formulating the idea that under the power of suggestion the mind may change the control of blood flow over specific spots in the body, so that strong substances may be released locally and may make one bleed or may stop the bleeding. My reaction can only be summed up as: Wow! Wouldn't such a specific control make sense in explaining why the hook-hangers in Sri Lanka or the fakirs in Mongolia and India do not bleed or tear their flesh? Wouldn't such a phenomenon explain why there was bleeding from the hands and feet of St. Francis of Assisi during religious ceremonies more than 700 years ago or from the palms of Father Pio Forgione in Forgia, Italy, who died in 1968, often displaying bleeding from sites similar to Jesus Christ's wounds?[30]

Hypnosis finally entered the realm of serious science in the 1950s, when remarkable findings started to emerge from the Stanford Laboratory of Hypnosis in the United States. Several amazing stories appeared in scientific journals, involving "automatic writing." As this term indicates, events that occur outside the subject's awareness can be recorded through the writing of the subject's hand under hypnotic suggestions. The hypnotized person, however, has no idea what the hand is writing. In 1957, G. H. Estabrooks reported an experiment with a friend who was reading *Oil for the Lamps of China* while his right hand, concealed behind a curtain, was holding a pen and was engaged in automatic writing on a pad of paper. The subject had been told under hypnotic suggestion that the hand would be out of his conscious awareness and no matter what happened to it, he would not feel any pain. Behind the curtain, Estabrooks pricked his friend's hand with a needle. The subject continued his reading while, behind the drape, the right hand "wrote a stream of profanity that would have made a top sergeant blush with shame" and even attacked

Estabrooks. Estabrooks commented that the subject was absorbed in his reading "without the slightest idea that his good right hand was fighting a private war."

It was not until 1974, however, that Dr. Ernest Hilgard proposed a theory on the mechanisms of hypnosis, reporting a ground-breaking experiment on a young woman who was an excellent subject, as she was hypnotized extremely easily and deeply. Her left arm was immersed in ice-cold water. As she had been told by suggestion that she would not feel any pain under hypnosis, she left her arm in the water with no signs of pain. Normally, one can endure freezing water temperature for only a few seconds or minutes before we would pull a blue hand out in great distress. The researchers had given this woman a pen and a pad of paper to write on. Guess what? Her right hand rated the pain in her left arm almost as high as if she were fully awake. In other words, a "hidden observer" within her own body was reporting pain, even if she felt no pain at all at conscious levels. Dr. Hilgard then proposed a new theory, called "neo-dissociation." He suggested that there is a split between a part of the older brain (in terms of evolution) that receives the noxious stimulus and recognizes it as harmful to the body, and the conscious brain (the part of the brain created more recently in human evolution) that the pain sensation does not reach. The woman's right hand records the pain that reaches the lower part of her brain, while her conscious mind remains oblivious to the painful stimulus and the pain.[31]

The bizarre phenomenon of "mind over matter" during hypnosis came up for discussion at the Royal Society of Medicine annual meeting in England in 1986. At this particular meeting, the scientists discussed the Hadfield and Moody experiences as well as the Hilgard experiments involving the hidden observer. Dr Patrick Wall, a hard-core neuroscientist, ended the meeting with these prophetic words: "If claims that one arm can be hot and the other cold under the influence of the mind can be supported scientifically, then this is revolutionary, and the whole concept of pain pathways as we know them, will have to be rethought." Over the years that followed this meeting, traditional scientists started exploring more seriously the depths of the brain and the mind-body interaction.

Today, hypnosis commands real respect from the scientific community. It is considered an altered condition or state of consciousness. It does make a person more prone to suggestions, modifies both perception and memory, and may change a number of physiological functions such as sweating or the tone of blood vessels, functions that are not under our conscious control.

Slowly but surely, we are gathering evidence that the power of the mind can indeed produce changes to specific parts of the body. Pain has a sensory component, an affective or emotional component relating to the unpleasantness of pain and a cognitive part relating to our thoughts. The hypnotist may make suggestions that specifically target the affective component of pain by turning unpleasant sensations into neutral or pleasant ones. Other suggestions may "disconnect" the bad sensation from the body. Hypnosis works through more than one mechanism. First, it suppresses pain by "splitting" consciousness into two levels. Pain is registered on one level but is blocked from reaching into our awareness, as the example of the "hidden observer" demonstrates. Hypnosis also activates special pathways in the spinal cord that block pain.[32] Finally, it selectively reduces the unpleasantness of the pain by changing the meaning of pain. Interestingly, hypnosis does not work by mobilizing the endogenous opioid system, unlike vigorous exercise, vaginal stimulation, electrical stimulation or acupuncture. Recent and remarkable imaging studies of the brain in subjects under hypnosis show clearly that hypnotic suggestions targeting the unpleasantness of a pain experience affect a certain part of the brain, while suggestions targeting the intensity of the pain experience affect another part of the brain.[33]

Hypnosis today has been applied to patients with all kinds of pain, from cancer, nerve injury, muscular and bone pain to pain in the absence of injury. Other techniques that seem similar but do not involve hypnosis, such as biofeedback relaxation, are also used now to teach patients how to modify biological processes, for example by changing the blood flow to the fingers under certain instructions and practice. These techniques, while they use the mind, are not hypnosis because they do not alter consciousness.

Another Painful Story—Priority and Perspective

To help my patients who suffer with chronic pain understand the concepts of distraction and attention, I use the concept of an imaginary filter with holes of a defined size to explain how the process of paying attention works. We all have this kind of "filter" in our brains. At any given moment our brain simultaneously receives many stimuli from the environment outside our bodies and from within us—noises, lights, smells, sensation of hunger, touch, vibration and so on. Then, it "scans" all these stimuli and tries to assign importance or significance to them in order of rank, allowing only the important ones to go through and attract our attention. Usually, this process will result in some form of action relating to the most important stimuli, while the "unimportant" ones will be ignored.

While I am explaining this to my patient (and often the spouse or relative who accompanies him or her to the office), I have my air conditioner working. The sound is light and constant, something between a hum and a purr, easily heard if one pays attention. All of a sudden I stop talking and ask the patient: "Do you hear anything in this room right now?" Now paying attention, the patient acknowledges that he or she can hear the air conditioning unit going. I then point out: "Well, when I was talking to you did you really notice the air conditioner?" Inevitably the patient had not noticed it. I continue: "That is exactly like what your mind was doing with me. Your brain considered what I was saying to you 'important' and worth paying attention to. At the same time, your brain deemed that the other sound in the room was 'insignificant' and just ignored it." I stress this concept by continuing with another example: "Let's imagine a mother and a baby. Their home is by the railway tracks. The train goes by regularly, shaking the house and filling the air with loud noise. The mother sleeps exhausted in her bed and does not even move despite all this racket and the vibration of the house. But when the little infant lets out a soft cry, she jumps out of bed to console her. In the mother's case, her brain labelled the baby's cry as 'significant' so the mother could take an action upon hearing it, while the train noise was 'insignificant,' therefore ignored."

My patients accept and fully understand the explanations. Then I link these examples with the way the brain views pain stimuli from injuries that have long since healed or insignificant lesions, like some arthritic changes within joints or some soft tissue/muscle strains, which still cause my patients agonizing pain. "These minor stimuli are now labelled 'important.' So they can go through your imaginary filter and reach your level of consciousness because you pay attention to them."

So far, so good. The patients typically respond: "Well then, Doctor, are you trying to tell me that my pain is all in my head?" I reply: "Exactly. All pain is in the brain, or to be exact, all pain perception is in the brain. If, for example, you need surgery for your appendix, your surgeon will put you under general anaesthesia. In other words, he or she will put your conscious brain to sleep, so you do not perceive the pain."

However, I explain, this does not mean that all stimuli from the body are to be ignored. Sometimes they are associated with significant local tissue changes and care has to be taken to address the local pathology. Other times, however, the original tissue damage is minor, but the stimuli from these body areas are still labelled "important" and go through, overriding others. When the patient is "hypervigilant" in detecting these stimuli and pays too much attention to them, some forms of treatment, such as behavioural-cognitive therapy, can be more effective than others, such as needles or medications addressing a physical problem or body site. Of course, in many instances, both things may happen: the tissue injury is sizable and treatable, and at the same time the attentional filter is supersensitive. In such situations, combined treatment approaches to both the physical and the psychological/behavioural aspects of pain are more effective.

The Placebo Effect and the Power of Suggestion

Anna was 74 years old, white haired and big hearted. I loved her smile the very first moment she came to see me for a consultation. Her orthopedic surgeon had sent her to me after he replaced her right knee with an artificial one. Anna continued to hurt profoundly, her knee was red and hot and she could neither touch the skin nor put her weight on that leg. The surgeon was wondering if she had reflex sympathetic dystrophy, a syndrome caused by dysfunction of the nervous system. I did not think so. Actually, I was quite worried that her knee was infected. I tried in vain to get in touch with the surgeon to find out what investigations he had done to rule out infection. He did not answer my calls. As there was no time to waste, I admitted Anna to my unit and ordered some specialized tests (bone scan and gallium scan) for her knee.

Anna was very happy with the care she was now receiving. She could not forgive the indifference of her surgeon and often referred to him with unflattering names. While waiting for the test results, I sent the physiotherapist to try to get Anna moving a bit. Long bed rest can bring numerous complications, such as blood clots, thinning bones and muscle wasting. Anna had not been active at all with this knee and had hardly gotten out of bed for two weeks.

Anna was with the physiotherapist as I entered the room. She had a big smile and she was taking little steps, supporting herself with a walker. The therapist had strapped a TENS (transcutaneous electrical nerve stimulation) machine around her knee to help a little with the pain. This machine delivers electrical impulses around the site of pain and may block certain types of pain messages.

"Wow," I exclaimed, "you seem to be walking well. How is your pain?"

"Very little, Doctor, very little. You guys seem to be doing amazing work here."

But the compliment did not impress me that much. Anna had a red, hot knee and I was almost sure it was infected. I had provided her with nothing much of a treatment except the little TENS machine, but I was not expecting such a response. If I was right and the knee was infected, how could she be having so little pain and be walking?

I decided to try a little test. I walked behind her while she was strolling slowly on her walker with no signs of pain . . . and squeezed her knee gently. She almost buckled. "You hurt me so much!" she cried.

That same afternoon the test results came back. Anna did indeed have a serious knee infection. I made rather urgent arrangements to have her transferred to another hospital with great expertise in the treatment of infected artificial joints. By the time the transfer was completed a few days later, the lower part of Anna's artificial knee had broken through the infected bone and was sticking out of her shin. Anna was operated on immediately, the knee prosthesis was thrown away and her knee was fused, as she was not going to be able to have a new prosthesis.

She phoned me a few weeks later from the rehabilitation hospital where she was recovering. "Doctor," she said, "I'm doing well now. I have a little shorter leg but they put a heel lift under my shoe. And you know what? The pain is gone now . . . for real."

This was one of my first encounters with the placebo effect. Anna had a true nociceptive problem with her knee. But when the therapist helped her get up and provided her with something she could see (the TENS machine), Anna was able to block her pain somehow and could walk. I say "somehow" because when I went behind her and squeezed that knee, pain reinvaded her consciousness. The infection was well established and her skin, muscle and bone nociceptors were quite irritated.

A placebo is "an ineffective treatment believed to be effective," and the placebo effect represents a "change in the patient's illness due to the symbolic significance of the treatment rather than pharmacologic or other physiologic effects of the treatment."[34] Good outcomes may be associated with ineffective or phony treatments as long as they are believed to be real. Placebo responses can occur with all kinds of treatments. These responses can vary: a placebo can relieve pain, wheezing, eliminate twisted posture or tremors, increase one's range of movement and do all sorts of things. Nearly 50 years ago a researcher named H. K. Beecher reviewed 15 studies of patients with different conditions, such as pain after surgery, coughing, angina, headache, mood changes, seasickness and anxiety.[35] He reported that the symptoms were relieved satisfactorily in 15 to 58 per cent of the patients across the different studies. Other studies have shown success rates with placebos as high as 70 per cent.[36]

In the past, many treatments were known to have high rates of good responses. Later, when these so-called beneficial interventions were tested and compared with sham or fake interventions, similar or better relief was obtained with the fake surgery or treatments. For example, 50 years ago, there was a popular procedure for the relief of heart pain (angina) in which the surgeons would open up the chest wall and tie a little artery inside the chest. This would result in dramatic relief in many patients. But when some surgeons decided to merely cut the skin open and then close it instead of tying up the artery, similar numbers of patients experienced significant pain relief.[37] Today, since Beecher's time, no drug is approved unless it has gone through exhaustive trials in which neither patients nor investigators know who is receiving the real drug and who is receiving an inactive, fake one. Unfortunately, we have accepted many surgical procedures today without similar comparisons for placebo effect.

One thing we physicians tend to forget is that suggestion can produce negative effects called *nocebo* effects, as well. In one study, 70 per cent of university students reported headaches when they were told that an electrical current was passing through their heads (which was not true).[38]

But why does the placebo effect occur? What accounts for the miraculous relief of spontaneous pain that Anna had, despite the florid infection in her knee? What accounts for the relief of pain obtained in so many studies with inactive drugs?

First, the expectations of the patient contribute to placebo analgesia. A positive attitude, anxiety levels, a willingness to abide by the treatment, a desire to get better, are all very important. At the same time, factors relating to those who offer the treatment are important too. Personal warmth, friendliness, the sympathy of the health care provider, as well as the prestige and reputation of the provider and the clinic or the hospital can all be significant. The appearance and the cost of the treatment also seems to count: red capsules seem to be more effective than yellow or white ones, needles are better than pills, and costly treatments have better results than cheap ones.

Placebos do more than just reduce anxiety or raise expectations. They have been shown to stimulate the release of endorphins.[39] The drug naloxone, which blocks endorphins, has been found to block the placebo effect in several studies. Lately, placebos have been found to produce respiratory depression, which was also blocked by naloxone. In other words, placebo-activated opioid systems act not only on pain mechanisms but on other systems as well. Furthermore, the activation of neurochemical systems by the sufferer expecting a good outcome goes beyond endorphins and beyond pain. For example, a recent study showed that in patients with Parkinson's disease, expectations of relief of tremor and rigidity after the administration of a placebo drug caused the release of endogenous dopamine (the specific chemical missing in this disease).

Anna liked my staff and my unit, and she also liked me. Besides, she deeply disliked her surgeon. She trusted us and expected she was going to get better in our hands. So, she managed to block her pain to a certain degree by subconsciously using the placebo effect and possibly by switching her attention as well . . . until my squeeze on the inflamed tissues gave her enough of a jolt to overcome her expectancy and her endorphins.

Getting better with a placebo does not necessarily mean "nothing is wrong with the patient." This is a serious misconception of both health care providers and patients. We are only scratching the surface in our efforts to understand pain relief under the power of suggestion during administration of placebos. Maybe in the future we as doctors will learn to use placebos to increase the good effects of medical treatments and decrease the bad ones, through release of the patient's internal opioids. A better understanding of the placebo mechanisms may provide new avenues to harness an individual's mental and chemical powers to his or her advantage.

Blocking My Own Pain

During the years that followed the birth of my first son, Nicholas, in 1985, and up to 1992, I suffered from back pain almost every day, the product of a seriously degenerated lumbar disc in combination with my lack of fitness. Provoked by certain encounters in my life, I set up a Nordic Track ski machine in one of my children's bedrooms in that crucial year of 1992. Slowly but surely I transformed myself into an avid fitness fanatic—I now train consistently many days every week, alternating between weightlifting and martial arts. Once the martial arts entered my life, my old pain parted but new and different pains appeared. Now, my newly found pains were infrequent but rather predictable visitors, which would attack knees, ribs, hamstrings, wrists and my back. Sometimes they would stay for days; sometimes they would persist for months. Amazingly, I befriended my pains, as I was often able to master them in ways I never knew before. While Jane's case had challenged my traditional medical knowledge early in my career, it was not until the appearance of my own pains—in the heat of a fight—that I became very much aware of how the human body (including mine) can completely block pain for certain periods of time.

My private lessons with pain came soon after I started training in tae kwon do, a form of Korean karate, in early 1996. Although I may have had strength and stamina, my lack of technique during contact fighting, called "sparring," was very much responsible for injuries that novices like me would sustain. One day, only six months into my training, I had to spar with an opponent much taller and heavier than I. Not only did Chris possess an exceptional physique, he had also been a trained martial artist for years. We were wearing protective gear—helmets, shin guards, gloves and *hogus,* a brace-like strong protective cover for the chest and upper abdomen. Feeling protected, we both exchanged a good deal of punches, jabs and kicks—true contact. Due to my lack of technique and experience, I found myself on the receiving end much more than Chris. It was not until quite later, maybe three-quarters of an hour or so, that I became acutely aware of a knife-like pain on my left side. I had finished the training, dressed and gone to pick up my car when the mere move to open up the car door with my left hand froze me right there in the middle of the street. I could not catch my breath. I knew then that I had done something to my ribs. By the time I arrived at my office, every deep breath and every twisting movement to do simple things like getting in and out of the car or even getting up from my office chair was accompanied by the same knife-like, breath-taking pain. Feeling my own rib cage, I came to the conclusion that I had cracked at least two ribs. To make matters worse, it was brought to my attention by a patient, hours later, that my left third toe was black and blue and sticking out sausage-like in my open-toed sandals. Examining this awkwardly swollen and deformed toe, I concluded that I had also cracked my toe, but I had felt no pain whatsoever until someone brought it to my attention. My office staff and my patients expressed no sympathy at all. My staff members kept giggling every time they heard me utter four-letter words in accompaniment to my efforts to bend over to examine a patient or simply rise from my chair. My assistant, Anna, announced emphatically that "she had no sympathy for people who submitted to self-abuse." My own patients would laugh at "a pain doctor who is in self-inflicted pain," as one lovely older woman told me. Four days later I was back in tae kwon do with some strong adhesive tape on my rib cage, but I restricted myself for a few days to movements and techniques that would not rekindle the pain from my healing fractures.

My inability to feel the acute pain upon impact when my bones broke, as well as the delayed onset of pain, surprised me, since I had never been exposed to situations like this before. But I was no different from the soldier in battle who does not feel the bullet until later, or the athlete in vigorous competition whose pain threshold is raised. Obviously the fight had taken sole possession of my attention. I certainly did not assign "unpleasantness" to the kicks, and I was under stress—good and wanted stress—which provoked release of my own endorphins.

One evening I was discussing the amazing stories of fakirs and hook-hangers with my husband Norm and my sons, explaining the endogenous analgesia system and endorphins, as well as the importance of attention and the necessity of unpleasantness in order to perceive pain as pain.

"Well," Norm said, "I had a very similar experience when I was young, maybe eight or nine years old. I was playing with my friends close to home. We were all climbing up on a shed and jumping down on the tall grass. On one occasion, as I landed on the grass I realized there was a pile of old lumber underneath. When I got up and attempted to walk away from the lumber, I felt something stuck under my shoe, as if I had stepped on a big piece of bubblegum. I looked down and saw a large plank nearly glued to the sole of my sneaker with a huge nail. For a moment I thought the nail was stuck to the thick rubber sole. I took a second look and . . . wow . . . I realized the nail had perforated the sole and my foot in the middle, sticking out above the top of the shoe! I had never felt any pain but I started screaming, more scared by the sight of the nail than from anything else. I walked home (about 30 metres, or 32 yards) screaming, still with no pain! Mom grabbed me and took me to the local emergency. The nurse pulled the plank off my shoe and my foot and took the sneaker off."

"So," I said, amazed by the story, "Was your shoe flooded with blood?"

"No. This was the strange thing. There was very little blood or anything, just a little red dot at the bottom of my foot and another one at the top, at the exit point of the big nail."

"Did you ever feel pain?" I asked.

"Yeah, big time—when the doctor made a fuss about the rusted nail and gave me a shot in the arm. That shot hurt me much more than the foot!"

Norm has no supernatural powers and has not trained his mind like the fakirs and the yogis. Simply, he was busy playing, his attention was consumed with the game and the friends and when the nail went through he did not feel pain and it did not tear his flesh (doesn't this sound so familiar?). It was the fuss of the medical staff about the rusted nail and the shot in the arm that hurt him more than the actual nail. Pain reached his consciousness only when his attention was directed to the arm and the foot.

All these examples of normal, everyday people like me, my family members and my patients, demonstrate how immense the power of the mind is and how little we know about these hidden forces within us.

Five

UNDERSTANDING PAIN

I saw Don some years ago, on the request of his family doctor. Don had fallen off a scaffold at work and had broken his right ankle. It was already two years after the injury when he came to my office, but he was still in bad shape. A torrent of complaints gushed out: "I am only 28 years old and I have pain every day. I can't walk without a limp, it hurts me the more I am up on my feet, and weather changes bother me so much that I feel like a barometer."

He said he felt a gnawing pain all the time. When stepping on the sore foot he would sometimes feel as though he was being stabbed in the ankle. The ankle itself was quite stiff; it made a peculiar cracking noise when I attempted to move it. Don looked irritable and his eyes got misty as he described how limited his activities were and how much he wanted to go back to work. But going back was hard for him, as Don was a waiter in a big restaurant, which meant that he had to be on his feet all the time.

Christian, 58, came to me with a long history of pain on the right flank, the part between his rib cage and his pelvis. He had seen a number of doctors until he was finally told that he had an unusually large right kidney. It contained cysts— bubbles filled with fluid. On several occasions, his doctors had inserted needles into these cysts, drawing out the fluid that was building under pressure. After every one of these sessions, Christian felt considerably less pain, but the effect was short-lived. The cysts would fill up again, stretching the lining of the kidney and bringing back intractable pain with each new stretching. Christian described his pain as deep pressure, as if something were going to explode inside his abdomen. He had to retire early from his job as manager in a retail mall and he was sad that he had not been able to enjoy playing with his grandchild.

Edward, the father of a colleague of mine, was a retired pharmacist who saw me about five months after a bizarre but devastating domestic accident. He was helping his wife Mildred prepare dinner in their Florida home. As Mildred was chopping meat the phone rang. She got to it at the same time as Edward. He extended his left hand to pick up the receiver, and within a split second his elbow hit the sharp edge of the knife in Mildred's hand. A quick scream, an electric jolt, a splash of blood and Edward's two last fingers went dead. Half an hour later in the local emergency room, the doctor told him that the knife had lacerated his ulnar nerve, a big nerve running under the "funny bone" in his elbow. This nerve is responsible for both sensation and certain movements in the wrist and fingers. By the time Edward came to see me, his left hand was shiny, the skin was paper thin, the fingers looked like sausages without the normal creases, and they were all very stiff. Edward could not make a fist. On top of this, he was unable to feel the touch of a Kleenex or the prick of a needle in these last two fingers. Edward described his pain as hot-burning, deep and shooting, waking him constantly at night. He was very distraught, as he was an avid golfer and was unable to play, let alone use his hand normally to make a fist or grab a fork. The pain was also getting worse when he attempted to keep his arm downward, swinging it during walking as we all do. Edward ended up with his hand in a sling.

Don, Christian and Edward had leg pains, tummy pains and arm pains respectively, yet they all shared certain common characteristics: chronic, intractable pain was interfering with their daily lives and had taken a stiff toll on their emotional well-being. Their pain had recognizable causes, in the sense that the pain was coming from specific types of injuries. Don had severe "post-traumatic arthritis" pain, as the fracture had gone through his ankle joint and damaged the cartilage and the bones. Christian's pain was produced by the stretching of the kidney capsule. Edward's came from the injured nerve that had set up a whole cascade of swelling, stiffness and diffuse aching, affecting not only the two fingers rendered useless by the lacerated ulnar nerve, but in fact his whole hand, and by extension, his arm. Unfortunately, Edward had developed a textbook case of "causalgia." This syndrome was first described in 1864 by Silas Weir Mitchell, a surgeon who treated injured soldiers in the U.S. Civil War. These unfortunate individuals would develop dreadful pains after gunshot wounds that damaged nerves in their arms or legs. Such pains could be so severe that some of the soldiers contemplated suicide.

In medical terms Don and Christian had developed "nociceptive" pain. This happens when the neurological structures that make up the *normal* pain system (receptors, nerve fibres and their connections with the spinal cord and the brain) become activated in skin, muscles, joints and abdominal viscera like the kidney and the bladder. Edward, by comparison, had developed "neuropathic" pain, which is the result of injury to the nerves, the spinal cord or the brain. This pain is now pathological pain, in the sense that it is a reflection of the *abnormal* functioning of the pain system.

The characteristics of nociceptive and neuropathic pain are quite different. Nociceptive pain can be divided into somatic and visceral nociceptive pain. *Somatic* means that the pain comes from muscles, tendons, bones and similar structures, while the term *visceral* refers to pain coming from organs within our chest and abdominal cavities (heart, lungs, stomach, gut, uterus, etc.). Fractures, sprains, strains, inflammation or infection of the joints or soft tissues all cause somatic nociceptive pain. Don's post-traumatic arthritis is that kind of pain. In such pains, local tissue injury activates the nociceptors, which in turn become sensitized. When this type of sensitization happens, these pain receptors tend to fire faster and at lower thresholds, so that pain can be caused by just a little stimulation, which normally would not be perceived as pain.

I know exactly what this means from personal experience. One time during heavy training, I was doing many crunches on the floor on an industrial rug in my martial arts gym. I felt a touch uncomfortable but it was not until I had a hot shower after the training, with the water splashing me, that I felt a painful burning sensation in my buttocks. Alarmed, I looked in the mirror and saw that I had a large area of peeled-off skin, leaving the flesh looking red and raw. I had sustained a "rug burn" because of the friction of my body on the hard rug. The nociceptors in this raw skin were now sensitized and they perceived the regular pleasant warmth of the water as very uncomfortable. Touching or pressing on the rug burn area gave me painful sensations.

This ultra-sensitive response to heat or touch or the prick of a needle is called *hyperesthesia,* and it is not unusual. Picture a patient with an inflamed joint because of gout. He has a big swollen "hot" toe that he cannot touch or move or squeeze. His nociceptors have received the message of the inflammation in the first place, sending painful signals to the brain, and these same nociceptors have become sensitized for as long as the inflammation lasts. The process is similar in the case of sunburn. Prolonged exposure to the sun will first make the skin turn reddish (for Caucasians, at least) before the body mobilizes the dye from the skin, called melatonin, that will change the red to a bronzy tan. During the first few days after a sunburn, the flesh is extremely sensitive. If you have ever experienced a bad sunburn—as most people of European descent have—even lying on the bed hurts and a warm shower is uncomfortable. But then the sensitivity subsides as our nociceptors normally "tune down" and return to their normal state. What we experience as the sunburn is healing is actually the typical reaction of a normally functioning pain system.

Such somatic nociceptive pains last as long as the inflammation or the tissue damage continues. We can pinpoint the part from which the pains originate, and these pains are frequently described as aching, throbbing, sharp or gnawing. Somatic nociceptive pains respond to anti-inflammatory (Aspirin-like) drugs and also respond well to morphine, which is much more powerful. But nociceptive pain that comes from deeper structures than the skin, such as muscles and bones, is confusing. A deep muscular pain can be a "dull" ache and may even be felt in a site far from the injury. This is called "referred" pain.

By comparison, a visceral nociceptive pain like the one that Christian feels from his kidney is quite different from a somatic pain. Our bodies contain different types of viscera—hollow ones like the bladder or solid ones like the liver and the spleen. Some years ago, experts believed that the viscera were impervious to pain—that they were unable to respond to violent, invasive stimuli such as cutting, crushing or burning. It is only in the last 20 to 30 years that we learned that viscera can indeed hurt, but such pains are different than the pains coming from muscles, bones and tendons. Visceral pains have specific characteristics. They are diffuse and poorly localized, they may produce local or whole body responses that are not very specific, they can raise our heart rate or blood pressure, they may cause skin and muscles over the ailing viscera to hurt and they can generate significant levels of fear or anxiety.

Visceral pain can be particularly ugly. When it's acute, for example when a kidney stone is lodged in the tube that connects the kidney with the bladder (the ureter), the pain comes in waves and can make one double over, feel nauseated and cause the heart to pound wildly. We know now that visceral pain can be caused by the stretching or contraction of the walls of hollow viscera, or in the case of Christian's kidney, the rapid stretch of the kidney "capsule." Other causes include lack of blood supply, inflammation of the lining of the viscera, distention and torsion or traction of the blood vessels of the viscera or the membranes that cover them in the abdomen. A remarkable property of visceral pains is their ability to create referred pains elsewhere in the body, pains that can be misperceived as coming from the skin, muscles or joints. Take for example the pain of angina or a heart attack, which often may radiate to the chest behind the breastbone, the jaw or the left arm.

The pain arising from injury or dysfunction of the nerves, the spinal cord or the brain is probably one of the hardest pains to treat and it is extremely difficult to understand. These neuropathic pains do not have the same characteristics as nociceptive pains and they usually do not respond to common treatments that would be recommended for arthritis, inflammation, muscle tears or fractures. Neuropathic pains can be experienced by patients whose nerves are damaged by diabetes, those who suffer from shingles or, as in Edward's case, after an injury to a large nerve. They can also arise when the nerve roots connected to the arm detach from the spinal cord (brachial plexus avulsion) or in cases of spinal cord injury or stroke. Such pains have many forms and shapes: they can be constant or may come abruptly and feel like electrical shocks or knife-like stabs. Anyone unfortunate enough to experience such pain might be unable to touch his or her skin, tolerate the breeze of a summer draft or the gently trickling water of a shower; it can hurt even to move the painful part. Often these pains are accompanied by changes in the appearance of the painful part—a swollen hand, a mottled foot, bluish hide-like skin, brittle nails. The limb may feel weak, stiff or cold and it may move involuntarily into a bizarre posture or start shaking.

In the vast majority of cases an injured muscle or tendon will heal well if the damage is not so severe as to create a lot of scar tissue. A broken bone will also heal as long as the broken ends are kept together and the limb is immobilized. But an injured nerve may never heal. Worse, an injured nerve often sets off a chain reaction. The site of the injured axon (the long arm of the nerve cell that carries messages from the tissue to the nerve cell itself) becomes supersensitive to minor movements of the body part. It also becomes supersensitive to certain chemicals circulating in our bodies, for example, adrenaline and noradrenaline excreted from our adrenal glands, a pair of little glands sitting on the top of our kidneys. Moving a hand to bring a fork to your mouth or grasping a glass of water will send ripples of abnormal messages from the injured site toward your spinal cord and brain. As if this were not enough, soon after a nerve injury, cells in the spinal cord that receive the abnormal messages from the part supplied by the injured nerve may start responding abnormally, as they become "sensitized." This sensitization is "central" because it occurs in the spinal cord, which is part of the central nervous system, as opposed to the sensitization of nociceptors after a sunburn or my own rug burn, which is "peripheral." The peripheral sensitization of nociceptors is a normal and common phenomenon in everyday events like cuts, burns, sprains and strains. Normally the healing process will result in elimination of peripheral nociceptor sensitization, as the pain system regains its balance. But central sensitization, which often follows a nerve injury, is very difficult to treat because it leads to a cascade of reactions. Each of these reactions at some point may acquire a life of its own, becoming independent from the injury that originally caused the problem.

Direct injury to the spinal cord or the brain (the central nervous system) creates what we call "central" pains (as opposed to peripheral neuropathic pains). Unfortunately, these kinds of central neuropathic pains are not easy to understand or treat. They can have the same bizarre characteristics of nerve injury pains (like sensitivity to touch, shooting and stabbing pains and so on).

Yet the cause of these central pains is found in cells within the spinal cord or the brain that fire on their own in bizarre ways or respond in completely abnormal manners to the messages coming from the skin, muscles or bones.

To make things even more complex, often we suffer with more than one kind of pain in combination. Nociceptive and neuropathic pains may interact, with bizarre outcomes and difficult symptoms that puzzle both the patient and the doctor. Even worse, intense pain mobilizes strong emotions, an incessant search to get rid of the problem, anxiety, worry, depression, anger and despair. And all these make our experience of pain more intense.

Treating Pain

Pain is such an integral part of everyone's lives. Tummy aches, headaches, nicks and cuts, toothaches, muscle pulls and sprains are everyday occurrences. The saving grace is that most of these come and go very fast. Acute pains create a strong drive to get rid of them. Some people do so by "toughing it out" and waiting for the pain to fade away, others will take over-the-counter medications. Some try local applications of remedies, such as hot packs, ice packs, ointments and creams. Sprains and muscle pulls or tight muscles (all somatic nociceptive pains) respond well to "hands-on" therapies by chiropractors, physiotherapists and massage therapists.

But is there any particular treatment that is "right" for everybody? Of course not. The treatment really depends on the type of pain, the location, the cause and the intensity—and that's just a start.

Visceral acute pains—things like menstrual pain, and gall bladder pains or the colic that results from a kidney stone—can be helped by the application of local heat through devices such as a hot water bottle or an electric heating pad. Sophisticated gadgets aren't necessary. I still remember an old woman, a neighbour of ours when I was a child in Greece, who used to heat up the clothes iron, wrap it in a towel and lay it on her flank during kidney stone episodes.

Often, though, heat is not the right thing to do for some kinds of pain. A hot iron certainly won't do the trick when it comes to heart pains like angina.

Special medications such as nitroglycerin preparations, usually placed under the tongue for quick absorption, open the arteries around the heart muscle to allow more blood to flow to the oxygen-starved heart.

As the complexity and persistence of certain pains increase, more complex treatments become necessary in chronic situations, usually in the form of combinations of drugs and non-drug therapies. Generally, if persistent pains from muscles, bones, joints or ligaments do not respond to over-the-counter medications, the doctor may prescribe other drugs such as muscle relaxants and strong painkillers. Another common treatment is the local application of "pain-relieving modalities"—hot and cold packs fit into this category, as well as more sophisticated machines operated by therapists, using lasers or ultrasound, that generate heat in deep tissue well below the skin. While hot and cold packs can work better for acute pains, other treatments are almost exclusively used to treat chronic pains, for example, electrical stimulation over the skin (transcutaneous electrical nerve stimulation, or TENS). This treatment involves the placement of electrodes or electrical wires over the skin of the painful part, connected to a small battery. Some forms of TENS can mobilize the body's natural endorphins and can be useful in alleviating nociceptive pains. Physiotherapists and kinesiologists can help too, by teaching exercises to increase the range of movement and the strength of muscles, or to help people correct their posture, balance and gait. Massage therapists work over muscles and tendon attachments and ligaments that may be tight or in spasm. Chiropractors use forms of quick oscillations in an effort to produce balanced action of muscles over joints and bones primarily along the spine. Other therapeutic exercise regimens such as yoga, Pilates and Feldenkrauss can help correct posture and strengthen and stretch muscles. It's also important to keep up with some sort of cardiovascular training—walking, working out on a treadmill or more sophisticated exercises.

Unfortunately, all of these various treatments just touch the tip of the iceberg, as chronic pain involves not only body parts, but also thoughts, feelings and emotions. Pain that lingers for weeks and months creates insomnia, anxiety, frustration and depression. That is why it is so common to see chronic pain patients who take handfuls of medications for ailments aside from their pain. Too many medications can be hard on the stomach, so the patients I see often need additional remedies for stomach upset or irritation. Strong painkillers containing some form of narcotic produce constipation, which will lead patients to supplement their diets with huge amounts of fibre or laxatives. Some of these patients have additional medical problems such as high blood pressure, high blood lipids or diabetes and heart or kidney disease; this means they need still more medication. In a chronic pain clinic like mine, patients often show up with bags full of pill bottles, which they then line up on my desk. Others simply bring a page with a long list of the medications they take. It's safe to say that not all patients understand why each medication is given, what kind of action and side effects each has and what kind of interactions take place when more than one medication is taken.

When it comes to treatment, neuropathic pains—Edward's type of pain—are not helped much by over-the-counter painkillers. They require stronger painkillers, such as codeine or morphine, alone or in combination with simple analgesics. In neuropathic pains the injured nerves "fire" abnormally; sometimes cells within the spinal cord and the brain cause pains by firing abnormally too. These nerves and cells may respond well to drugs that are otherwise used by people who suffer from epilepsy. There is a connection here. During a seizure, a part of the brain "fires" abnormally, as the cell membranes within the region of the brain that generates the epileptic seizure are unstable. Anti-epileptic drugs stabilize these irritable membranes to prevent seizures. They do the same thing to the injured nerve areas.

Tricyclic antidepressants are a special class of drugs used to fight depression. They can also work as a first-line defence against neuropathic pain, and they can treat some forms of headaches and may help with sleep. My patients are often taken aback when I propose these drugs, wondering why I recommend them since they do not feel depressed. I then explain that these drugs can also work to combat some kinds of chronic pains.

The truth is that there are many therapies one can offer to patients with chronic pain, but no one therapy or drug works well for all patients. Drugs may work in some cases; in others, stress management or even psychotherapy or a cognitive-behavioural program might help. Blocking particular nerves, injections, surgery to cut down neural tissue and even implanting electrical stimulators in nerves, the spinal cord and the brain, are all techniques that have their place. Most often, treatments that address the physical and the emotional aspects of the pain experience together work much better than just one form of treatment alone.

Chronic pain means persistent pain for months and years. Conventional medical wisdom holds that if you have pain that lasts less than six months you are in "acute pain." If your pain lasts longer, it is chronic. Personally, I think this is simplistic—and troublesome, as chronic pain cannot simply be defined only by its duration. There are additional characteristics that distinguish acute and chronic pains. For example, most of the time, acute pain has a specific source—a broken bone, a sprained ligament, inflammation and so on. Acute pain will also invade the entire body. A kick in the groin will raise blood pressure and make the heart race and cause the victim to gasp for air, sweat, scream and suffer muscle spasm—it's not just the groin that recoils in agony. When the cause of acute pain is removed, these body reactions disappear too. In contrast, as the pain becomes "chronic," the changes in heart rate, breathing or blood pressure or the reflex spasms tend to get minimized, while emotions and thoughts get more complex and intense.

Chronic pain is not the same as "chronic pain syndrome" or "chronic pain disorder." These terms are often used interchangeably; that is a mistake that can make things extremely confusing for patients, doctors, insurers and courts. A patient with chronic arthritis of the hip, for example, hurts almost every day, especially after standing for long periods, or when the weather changes. But typically the patient still goes about, doing as many things as possible, and maintaining a grip on life and personal relationships. This patient, as far as I'm concerned, has "chronic pain."

By contrast, when the pain "gets on our nerves," it moves into "chronic pain disorder" territory. In such cases, persistent pain can distort one's personality, change one's physical functioning and social interactions, and alter the way one thinks about the world when one gets up in the morning. Yet in most cases of chronic pain disorder, what remains of the original physical injury may be quite insignificant. The more you move toward emotional decompensation in the face of chronic pain—that is, the more your emotions "go down the drain"—the more difficult the situation becomes. Chronic pain disorder or syndrome can lead to high levels of disability—the feeling that you just can't function properly anymore. It has to be addressed from multiple fronts, as the emotional side effects and dealing with the sufferer's friends, relatives and colleagues and their reactions, are significant issues. The physical problem can often be the least important aspect to treat.

I think it's a serious misconception on the part of treating physicians or health care providers to believe that chronic pain disorder is not present unless six months have gone by. Studies show that workers with soft tissue injuries who are away from work for just a bit more than four weeks are at risk of developing long-term disability and chronic pain disorder and they should be treated early with intense multidisciplinary rehabilitation techniques.[1] These types of programs address function as well as emotional and physical well-being in a concerted approach, with the help of many professionals (physicians, psychologists, physiotherapists, social workers and others). Treating chronic pain syndrome means more than just looking at the physical symptoms. There is also much emotional, behavioural and social damage that needs to be repaired.

Six

MUSCLES AND BONES, SUCCESS AND FAILURE

One day during my rounds at the hospital a colleague, Larry, came up to me. "I've got a problem," he said. "My wife and I went shopping 2 days ago and when I bent over to lift a couple of cases of Coca-Cola, I got this sharp pain at the left side of my back. It is a little better now but it still hurts quite a bit and I can't seem to get comfortable at all. Over the last three years I've had a couple of episodes like this, lasting 7 to 10 days each time."

A lot of people will recognize this situation. In any case, I offered to examine my colleague. Larry was 36, a father of two and very busy as a doctor and scientist. He was living a sedentary life, spending endless hours in the office or at the computer, getting exercise only from the occasional stroll or from gardening. Although he was not overweight, he was clearly out of shape. He had a protruding belly and his head was thrust forward while his shoulders were rounded, all signs of poor posture and poor physical condition. He pointed to the left side of the small of his back. As I examined him, except for his limited ability to bend or stretch his back because of pain, I noticed that he was stooped forward and to the left. I felt under my fingers a hard, rope-like structure on his left side that was very tender; it was a bunch of back muscles, tight like a knot. I looked at his spinal X-rays and they showed very little. There was nothing else in my examination to indicate any serious problem. If he had complained of leg pain and he had changes in his reflexes, muscle strength or sensation, I would have been worried about a herniated disc.

Backache is such a frustrating symptom, for the doctor as well as for the patient. The spine is not a mere supporting pillar of our bodies; it is vital in our ability to walk and move from one point to another. It is this function of the spine, and the flexibility it requires, that leads to many causes of backache. A body part that is in use so much of the time inevitably will suffer stress and show signs of abuse if we are not careful. It is a misconception that humans have back problems simply because they have been standing on their legs in an erect posture as opposed to our ancestors, the apes. The reality is that humans have stood erect for at least five million years but we have been plagued by back pain only in the last 10,000 years—a time that corresponds to our habit of picking things up and carrying them around.[1]

In Larry's case, his rather weak abdominal muscles and poor posture plus his inappropriate lifting techniques were responsible for the pulled muscles or ligaments that I thought he suffered from. Since he had suffered similar episodes before, he was worried that there would be more to come. He was quite right to be concerned. As we get older, the discs (the little cushions between the vertebral bodies, the bones of our spines) lose part of their water content and become weaker and thinner. Similarly, the little joints at the back of the vertebral bodies, called facets, may suffer from arthritic or degenerative changes. Finally, the ligaments that support the spinal column may get stretched and weak. Recurrent back pain like Larry's can lead to chronic pain, particularly when disc, facet and ligament changes are added.

I wish I'd had some magic advice for Larry, but I didn't. I prescribed a simple course of non-steroidal anti-inflammatory drugs (aspirin-like drugs), suggested he use a hot pack for 20 to 30 minutes at a time and most importantly, I sent him to our physiotherapists to teach him a back exercise and education program.

I warned him that if he wanted to avoid recurrent episodes and chronic pain, he had no other option but to strengthen his abdominal muscles through regular exercise, to learn how to bend and lift properly and to get engaged in a general fitness program. I painted a bleak future of back pain recurrences if he did not leave his "couch potato" attitude and I gave him a bit of a pep talk. I stressed that he was still a young man, that he had many more years to live and that he had better live them by doing his best to avoid chronic or recurrent pain. To make the point that there is a limit to what I, or anyone else, can do, and that it is solely up to him to take his back care into his own hands, I reminded Larry of the old Groucho Marx joke:

> Patient: "Doctor, Doctor, after the surgery am I going to be able to play the violin?"
> Doctor: "I hope so."
> Patient: "Good, because I could never play it before."

I must have either scared or impressed Larry enough for him to decide to take his back pain seriously: soon he started taking long power-walks at least three times per week and began a program of regular muscle stretching. As the months passed, I noticed that he had lost some weight and his tummy looked flat. Eventually, he moved to another hospital, but I still see him once in a while. Once when we met, Larry told me proudly that he "kissed his back pains goodbye" and had never had any other episodes once his fitness and lifestyle regimens changed.

I couldn't be more delighted. And I knew exactly what he meant. I too had lived with chronic recurrent back pain for eight years. I had a lot more going wrong with my back than Larry (including a narrow and degenerated disc and shut facet joints at the lower part of my spine), but I also shared the common "couch potato" attitude and lived by the "don't-have-time-for-exercise" mantra. Once I changed my lifestyle and fitness became an integral and necessary part of my life, I kissed my pain goodbye as well, even though my back has already undergone significant degenerative changes.

Tom's story is quite different. Tom, a 34-year-old friend of mine, was an extremely busy financial planner but he always found time to exercise. He was an avid cyclist and had a home gym with state-of-the-art equipment and a personal trainer who would train him at 6 a.m. three times a week for at least an hour. He was fit and slim, a real "exercise freak." However, one day while performing his heavy squats with several plates of weight on his back, he experienced a searing pain in the right side of his lower spine, radiating down to his right leg. He phoned me in agony and I stopped by to see him at his home after I finished work. He was in a fair amount of pain, his back muscles were tender and tight, and on examination I noticed that he had a patch of numbness at the outside of the right foot, while he had lost what we doctors call his ankle jerk. Tendon jerks are generated when the doctor hits your ankle joint (knee, elbow or wrist) gently with a reflex hammer at the point where the tendon is attached. When the limb reacts with a kick, it tells the doctor that the nerves that supply the tendons and muscles of these joints are intact.

It was clear that Tom had a herniated disc. A herniated disc occurs when the jelly-like inner content of the disc, which is shaped like a doughnut, escapes partially to the outside through a tear of the fibrous ring that forms the outer layer. This extruded disc material then exerts pressure on the surrounding nerves and is responsible for the muscle spasms, the back pain, the radiating leg pain and the changes in reflexes and sensation down the leg. All of these symptoms are commonly known as sciatica, because the sciatic nerve at the back of the thigh is the one that is affected most of the time in the low back. Most herniated discs shrink back within a few weeks. Strong painkillers and local application of a hot pack, maybe a couple of days of rest, progressive and gradual mobilization followed by abdominal strengthening programs and gradual return to regular physical activities are sufficient in the vast majority of cases to make the pain and weakness go away within weeks. But Tom was neither that lucky nor patient enough to wait.

When his excruciating pain had continued for a week, I organized a CAT scan (which is what was available at the time, in the early 1990s) and a consultation with one of the neurosurgeons on my team. Tom ended up having a quick surgery soon after, a procedure called a microdiscectomy. The neurosurgeon opened up a small incision at the small of his back, about 2.5 centimetres (an inch), and used a microscope to "fish" out the herniated disc fragment. It turned out that Tom had more than a simple herniated disc. He actually had what we call a "sequestered" disc, where the disc fragment gets completely detached from the disc body and dislodges itself onto the surrounding structures and nerve roots. Most herniated discs will respond to non-surgical management, but a stray piece of disc will usually require surgery. It worked for Tom— he went home the second day after the surgery and gradually and carefully resumed his fitness activity during the next three months. To this day, Tom continues to bicycle and exercise regularly, retaining his slim physique, but he had to reduce his weightlifting and monitor carefully what he does. He still has the odd muscle strain but other than that he is doing very well and leads an active lifestyle.

Larry and Tom are not typical of the patients who visit my pain clinic. Their problems are more straightforward and could be managed by the family doctor or, as in Tom's case, by a neurosurgeon. Back pain is an extremely common medical problem and seems unavoidable for most of us as we get older. It is indeed one of the most common reasons for visiting the family physician and the most frequent cause of disability for workers younger than 45.[2] Low back pain is responsible for 20 per cent of all industrial injuries and accounts for nearly half of the costs of all these injuries. Ten per cent of the back injuries sustained at work become chronic and account for an astounding 80 per cent of the money spent by workers' compensation boards to cover time off work, permanent disability and medical costs. Acute low back pain, however, is short-lived in the vast majority of sufferers; in nine out of ten people, an episode of low back pain like the one Larry experienced will limit activity for less than 30 days. Of those with acute low back pain who do seek medical care, 25 to 40 per cent may have symptoms that look like sciatica, but only 2 to 5 per cent will have actual neurological signs—change in reflexes, strength and sensation—as Tom experienced. Even among those few who show neurological symptoms and signs that suggest disc herniation, half will recover enough within 30 days, so that they don't require surgery.

Low back pain is nearly unavoidable for most of us by age 50, but the severity and intrusiveness varies extensively. Unfortunately, the treatment and understanding of low back pain has been characterized for many years by irrational approaches. One such irrational approach is the use of screening X-rays. They rarely give additional information beyond what can be extracted by a good history and physical examination. Another wrong assumption is that degenerative changes that show up on X-rays, CAT scans or MRIs mean that something is "wrong" with our back. In reality, when the history and physical examination do not indicate that something is truly wrong, X-ray findings should be ignored. A 50-year-old *without* any symptoms whatsoever has a 50 per cent chance of abnormal findings in a lumbar spine CAT scan or MRI, and a 70 per cent chance of abnormal spinal X-rays, showing some disc degeneration or arthritic changes. As we get older, the appearance of certain abnormalities in radiological tests has no more significance to the body than the greying of our hair. However, we don't go to the doctor to treat grey hair (the hairdresser does a better job anyway).

Epidemiologists tell us that back problems have come to be considered a medical disability issue in the Western world only in the last 50 years or so, when back pain evolved "from being a part of life to classification as an injury for worker's compensation and insurance purposes."[3] By contrast, in developing societies such as Oman, the Ivory Coast and Nepal, back pain is considered a part of normal life. In these countries, major afflictions such as polio are quite prevalent and can generate back pain because of weakness and unbalanced gait. The pain, however, seems to be much less debilitating for individuals or for society there compared with how people suffer in the West.[4]

What kinds of people develop intractable pain that leads to serious disability? Who are the patients who end up visiting a pain clinic like mine again and again? I believe I gained some insights into this early in my career from my encounters with a patient I'll call Bruno.

He was 36, working in construction as a drywall installer. Bruno's family doctor sent him to me nine months after he had injured his back at work. Acupuncture and simple painkillers did not seem to work. By the time I saw Bruno, he limped and stooped over, with his hand always at his back, and he told me in colourful terms how severe his back pain was. His sleep was disturbed, he had a fair number of arguments with his wife, as he was able to do very little at home, and he had put on weight and looked depressed. I realized that the therapy he had been given early in his problem was "passive," meaning that the therapist was doing things *to* him as opposed to helping him learn active exercises and start a fitness program. I put him on tricyclic antidepressants, good for his sleep, his low mood and his chronic pain, and I sent him to a local physio-therapy department with a prescription for "active" physiotherapy.

But Bruno did not get much better.

My attempts to return him to the workplace were unsuccessful. His employer was not particularly willing to give him a lighter job. Bruno stayed as my patient for about a year and a half and then he disappeared. He returned for a visit some years later, still out of work, tangled in dispute with the Workers' Compensation Board, separated from his wife, depressed and on social assistance.

In retrospect, I realize I failed to recognize some important signs—signs that contributed to Bruno's chronic pain disorder and his disability. For one thing, it turned out that he had a previous history of two back injuries that had kept him out of work for months at a time. But that was not all. Bruno had little educa-tion and limited work skills, as well as a difficult, unsympathetic employer whom Bruno did not particularly like. Today, workers' compensation boards have become much more aggressive in dealing early with soft tissue and other injuries and pain. In these circumstances, Bruno would have qualified quickly for an intense functional restoration program that may have helped him more. The primary goal of these types of programs is to restore the patient's function, with the hope that as the function improves, pains decrease as well. In my own jurisdiction of Ontario, such programs involve five to six weeks of intense, multidisciplinary psychosocial rehabilitation, with both physical conditioning and mental and behavioural training in how to cope with and reduce pain. Counsellors from such programs would have provided Bruno with "work hard-ening" to prepare him to return to employment, and they would have visited Bruno's employer to work out a suitable schedule and duties for his attempt to return to work.

Bruno is one kind of back pain patient who frequents my clinic. Victor is another. At 47, Victor had several back surgeries after a fall at work as an engi-neer with an airplane manufacturing company. When he was diagnosed with sciatica, his surgeon operated on him within two months. I read this doctor's surgical notes and realized that except for a bulging disc, the quick-to-operate surgeon did not find much else. Victor did not get that much better.

In fact, within six months he got worse. He started to feel numb and tingly in his right leg, in addition to the pain he suffered since before the surgery.

After some tests, the surgeon opened him up again to find a fair amount of scar tissue formed after the first operation, encasing a couple of nerve roots. He cleaned up the scar tissue, giving Victor a few months of improvement until . . . the pain came back viciously, both in the back and the leg. Victor searched for another surgical opinion and he ended up with another surgeon and another surgery. This time it was a back fusion, an operation in which the surgeon places a chunk of bone and usually some hardware (rods or pins or plates) in between two or more vertebral bodies to "fuse" them together so that they do not move.

When the third surgery did not work, Victor visited my clinic. By that time he was in serious pain (mostly in his lower back, less in his leg) and he was depressed, complaining that his life at home was hell and thinking all the time of suicide. I prescribed a number of medications—anti-epileptics to control the neuropathic pain in his leg, antidepressants (in this case, for his depression) and morphine—and sent him for stress management and counselling. Victor's quality of life improved enough so he was able to see easier days and to lead a better family life. His pain was brought under enough control to allow him to enjoy a few things he used to do before, take some correspondence courses and even spend a couple of afternoons a week in a community centre doing volunteer work. But he was unable to return to work as he would have liked. Victor was suffering from "failed back syndrome" (also known as "failed back surgery syndrome"), an all-inclusive term referring to persistent back pain after all kinds of treatments, usually including one or more back operations.

In the United States, more than 300,000 spinal operations are performed each year (more than in any other Western country) with *10 to 40 per cent* of those leading to failed back syndrome.[5] Failed back syndrome originally was associated with open surgery, but new ways of tampering with the spine have added new categories of treatment failures. Failed back syndrome can even occur after procedures in which the surgeon does not have to "open up" the back, such as percutaneous discectomies (destroying a disc by inserting needles rather than through a true surgical incision) and chemonucleolysis (injecting chemicals like chymopapain that "eat away" the herniated disc). The warning "no matter how severe or intractable the pain is, it can always be made worse by surgery" should always be kept in mind.[6]

But what accounts for such an astonishing failure rate? The most common causes are choosing the wrong patient for surgery and making the wrong diagnosis.[7] In other words, what was wrong with the patient could not be fixed with surgery, and the surgeon should not have offered an operation in the first place.

Sometimes surgery will make no difference because there is already permanent nerve damage, caused by direct and irreversible injury to the spinal roots because of persistent compression by a herniated disc. This is the second most common cause of failed back syndrome. This is why it's so important to have the right diagnosis: significant disc herniation with persistent root compression should not be left untreated for more than six months.[8]

A less common cause of persistent pain after a back operation is incomplete surgery. It may be that the surgery did not take out all the disc material or remove extra bones that could be compressing nerve roots. Surgery can also create new problems, such as making segments of the spine unstable; causing new damage to nerves, muscles and bones; accelerating degenerative changes; and forming scar tissue or causing inflammation of the linings of the spinal roots (nerve root fibrosis or arachnoiditis).[9]

When failed back syndrome occurs, most patients like Victor will need referral to a multidisciplinary pain program similar to mine, as they suffer not only physically but also mentally and emotionally. Victor was a textbook case: his surgeon was quick to operate for no good reason, surgery gave him additional complications with scarring of the nerve roots, and his third surgery, the back fusion, gave him additional problems and more arthritis in the disc spaces above the fused part of the spine.

Surgery for low back pain is rarely indicated. Most patients will respond to non-surgical treatments. If both the physical and non-physical components of low back pain are addressed in a wise and reassuring manner, most back pains will ease. Conditioning, education and early introduction of gradual activity are the cornerstones of management for most cases of low back pain. Surgery should be considered only in a few cases, and even then only after a two- to six-month trial of non-surgical management.

Bruno's and Victor's chronic low back pains, which are difficult for doctors to treat, are not the only kind of chronic pain that puzzles physicians and make them send their patients to clinics like mine. Chronic pain affects a large part of the Canadian population. An older study has suggested that chronic pain affects 10 per cent of Canadians. A more recent study raises the numbers even more— nearly one in five Canadians over the age of 15 have chronic pain, according to the most recent National Population Health Survey (1996–97).[10] The numbers are similar in the United States and other Western nations. This percentage increases considerably as we get older—how many of us do *not* know someone of middle or advanced age who has chronic pain from arthritis, or complications from diabetes or shingles? Still, despite the millions of us who suffer, doctors do not fare well when it comes to managing patients with chronic pain. A recent survey of Ontario physicians showed that the burden of chronic pain management lies primarily on the shoulders of primary care physicians; clinics like mine get referrals of the truly hard-to-treat cases, those which haven't responded to traditional pain management in the family doctor's or specialist's office.[11]

Helen was one such case. She was 37 when she first saw me. She had been suffering from headaches since her mid-20s. In the beginning, her headaches were typical migraines, always localized to one side of the head, once or twice per month. They were serious and throbbing; she felt sick to her stomach. She preferred to retreat to a dark and quiet room until the migraines went away, usually within a day. She had tried several medications and, in particular, she had been helped by a drug called Imitrex that she used to take at the onset of headaches. She did well for years, holding a full-time job, until the pattern of her headaches changed dramatically, about six years before her referral to me.

By the time I met Helen, her headaches would start slowly and spread throughout her head, lasting up to five days. She no longer felt nauseated when she had a headache, and Imitrex had stopped working. At the same time as the headache pattern changed, Helen noticed that her upper and lower back started bothering her, and later she developed knee pains as well. By the time she came to see me, she had made the rounds of chiropractors who told her that her back was out of place, rheumatologists who diagnosed her as having fibromyalgia (diffuse soft tissue pain of unknown cause), and anaesthetists who gave her many injections into the muscles of her head, neck and back. Her family physician had also placed her on many cocktails of medications, with little pain relief. Little attention, however, had been paid to Helen's personal life.

It turned out that Helen's boyfriend had left rather unexpectedly after several years of a relationship. Shortly after, Helen found out that he was dating another woman. She fell into deep depression for which she had to be hospitalized. It was then that her diffuse, debilitating headaches started, followed by several other body pains. Because of her chronic pains she was unable to keep her job and in the end she went into long-term disability. She became isolated as her friends slowly disappeared. By the time she saw me, she was more or less housebound, using large doses of strong pain medications like morphine with little relief. Obviously Helen had not recovered from her deep hurt and anger over the failed relationship, and she hadn't looked for psychological counselling, as she insisted that her pains were all physical. But my team, which includes a psychologist and a psychiatrist, agreed that unless Helen faced up to her emotional turmoil and ended her isolation, which contributed to the tension in her back, neck and face, we would not be able to improve the headaches.

We made arrangements for her to see a psychologist close to her home and to attend a program of chronic pain management and biofeedback-relaxation. Biofeedback-relaxation involves the placement of electrodes over the face and upper back muscles, picking up signals of increased muscle tension. The patient can hear a distinct sound and see lines on a screen representing the activity of the hyperactive and tight muscles. By becoming aware of the excessive muscle activity through her ears and eyes, then, she could learn to try to relax the muscles consciously. We also suggested that Helen drop some of her ineffective and addictive medications. We were not against her using drug therapy, just inappropriate drug therapy. We added some strong antidepressants and we made arrangements for her to be involved in some volunteer community work. Did all this help Helen? Unfortunately, no. Her long-term disability insurance would not pay for psychological treatment and biofeedback-relaxation and Helen could not afford it, so what we recommended was never carried out.

Nevertheless, I think our team approach was the right one. Helen's problems were complex and called for an eclectic array of treatments. She had also been diagnosed as suffering from fibromyalgia, a diagnosis that is given very frequently to patients who "hurt all over." Fibromyalgia is a puzzling disease with an unknown cause—one of several new, chronic conditions of undetermined origin, such as chronic fatigue syndrome, repetitive strain injury and environmental sensitivity that have appeared during the last 20 to 40 years.

The sufferers of fibromyalgia complain of diffuse muscle pain, often accompanied by fatigue, disturbed sleep, morning stiffness, headaches, irritable bowel syndrome and other debilitating symptoms. The characteristic diagnosis is made when the patient is found to have 11 or more tender points out of 18 in total, located in specific sites. For years researchers have tried to find a reason for the constellation of these symptoms, but so far they have failed to discover a specific physical or psychological cause.

One of the most recent books I read on the subject gives me goosebumps. *Under the Medical Gaze*[12] is the personal story of Susan Greenhalgh, an anthropologist at the University of California, who was diagnosed as suffering from fibromyalgia by a rheumatologist. In this remarkable book of personal emotions and passion intertwined with extremely well-researched scientific and other literature, Susan presents her encounters with a specialist who used the established diagnostic criteria for this newly emerging disease and who convinced both himself and his patient that she had this painful muscle condition, which is often thought to be untreatable. She describes her eight-month experience with the diagnosis of fibromyalgia, the way conventional medicine takes labels and turns them into physical disorders necessitating dramatic life changes and drugs, her compliance with medical treatments, her desperate journey toward alternative and New Age medicine that only led her to fall deeper into despair and illness, and finally her rebellion against the diagnosis and overmedicalization of the problem.

Fibromyalgia scarcely existed in 20-century literature as a disease in its own right until 1977, when two Canadian doctors, Harvey Moldofsky and Hugh Smythe, published a paper that laid down criteria for the diagnosis of what at the time they called "fibrositis."[13] The paper generated tremendous interest in the condition, and an editorial in the *Journal of the American Medical Association* in 1987 described fibromyalgia, a name most scientists preferred to fibrositis, as a common cause of pain. Finally, a committee set up by the American College of Rheumatology published the definition and diagnostic criteria of the syndrome in 1990.[14] After this, fibromyalgia was really on a roll. It is estimated today that a considerable number of adults (2.4 per cent of the general population and 20 per cent or more of all patients visiting a rheumatologist) suffer from fibromyalgia, with women affected seven times more often than men.[15]

Soft tissue pain is a substantial problem. Some doctors believe that the diffuse soft tissue pain of fibromyalgia is distinct from other types of localized soft tissue pain (called myofascial pain), which seem to be associated with specific "trigger" points. However, epidemiological studies provide evidence that fibromyalgia is not a separate disease, but rather part of a spectrum of chronic pain phenomena in which there is soft tissue tenderness. Contrary to the belief of many that fibromyalgia is a lifelong disorder with no specific or permanent cure in sight (a truly depressing prospective that leaves the sufferer lost and hopeless), studies show that diffuse or localized soft tissue pains have a variable course and outcome. A group of patients visiting family doctors were studied twice, at the beginning of the study and 12 months later. The researchers found that those patients who had widespread pain at the start of the study were more likely to continue with widespread pain a year later, but this was not an inevitable path. For more than a third of the patients the pain had shrunk to one area only, and 18 per cent were completely free of pain.[16] In other words, approximately half those studied were at least better after a year.

The relationship between chronic soft tissue pain and trauma is an open and troublesome issue from both the medical and legal point of view. About 10 per cent of all women with no complaints of pain whatsoever will have 10 or more tender points, while 11 to 18 tender points are necessary for the diagnosis of fibromyalgia. Keeping in mind that a range of tender points occurs "naturally" in the general population, if a patient after a traffic accident is found to have tender points, there is a 1 per cent chance in men and a 10 per cent chance in women that the tender points were there before the accident.[17] Another piece of evidence against the concept of fibromyalgia as a specific disease entity comes from a worrisome statistic. In a study conducted by one of the "fathers" of fibromyalgia, Hugh Smythe, the doctor and his team had difficulty telling who had real pain and who was faking: 15 per cent of patients with diffuse pain were thought to be "fakers," while a whopping 10 to 40 per cent of those who *actually* faked pain were mislabelled as having fibromyalgia.[18] This outcome certainly speaks volumes about the lack of specific diagnostic criteria for fibromyalgia.

An important question relates to the actual costs of disability when it comes to soft tissue pain. Over the past two or three decades, we have seen a flurry of terms or labels for poorly understood chronic conditions such as fibromyalgia, fibrositis, myofascial pain, chronic pain syndrome, chronic fatigue syndrome, myalgic encephalomyelitis, nonarticular rheumatism, psychogenic rheumatism, repetitive strain injury and who knows what else. The names may vary, but all these conditions share common characteristics: they have persistent soft tissue pain, an obscure relationship to a specific injury, unknown or mysterious mechanisms responsible for the symptoms, and problems correlating what is physically wrong with the degree of the person's disability or distress.

What do these newly emerging diseases cost? When London Life of Canada conducted a review of long-term disability (LTD) claims and the results were extrapolated to all LTD carriers in this country, the following astounding figures emerged: Group LTD carriers paid out $46 million for fibromyalgia claims, $30 million for repetitive strain injury claims and $27 million for chronic fatigue claims in 1994 alone![19] Costs like these cannot help but influence the attitude of the public, the health care providers and the legal profession toward these chronic pain diagnoses.

My good friend and highly respected colleague Dr. Eldon Tunks from the Chedoke McMaster chronic pain management program in Hamilton, Ontario, has wondered whether some cases of chronic soft tissue pain such as myofascial pain, fibromyalgia or repetitive strain injury are not due more to an "intolerance to repetitive movements" than to actual muscle and soft tissue injury, at least in people who have multiple tender points. Maybe one's job, an injury or even more subtle factors "unmask" or aggravate this previously silent trait.[20] This concept makes a lot of sense to me. It leads me to additional questions about the relationship between the mind, pre-existing conditions in the body and the effects of a sudden change in conditions. What if these unknowingly vulnerable and tender people get involved in an accident that also creates emotional distress? What if the combination of emotional and physical acute trauma, added to the background of tender points, changes the way pain reaches consciousness and in turn leads to a change of the brain's activity and even more sensitivity to pain?

Today researchers around the world are investigating a huge number of factors that could possibly account for fibromyalgia. For some patients the disorder creates only minor inconvenience, but for others it is truly incapacitating.

Studies have looked at one extreme of the spectrum, a purely biomedical point of view (dysfunction of the body's metabolism, viral infection, immune system dysfunction, genetic predisposition, nervous system dysfunction and so on), to the other extreme, a psychological angle, (stress, sexual abuse, victimization and psychological dysfunction). Abnormalities have been found on both fronts but they are not specific or clear enough to define the syndrome as a distinct entity.

As a lifelong student of chronic pain, I have had a hard time accepting fibromyalgia as a specific, definable and hopeless entity, and I am not alone. This is not to say that it does not exist, or that I am insensitive to the suffering of those bearing the diagnosis. I simply feel that the diagnosis is given indiscriminately to too many people, and that all the symptoms attributed to fibromyalgia do not necessarily constitute a condition that is scientifically specific. My opinion is supported by the fact that the same constellation of symptoms is diagnosed as a different disorder by different specialists. For example, what rheumatologists call fibromyalgia, gastroenterologists label as irritable bowel syndrome, physiatrists (specialists in physical medicine dealing with disability after diseases or injuries) know as myofascial pain syndrome and psychiatrists name as hypochondriasis. The vast array of symptoms shared in all these overlapping disorders makes none of them specific, unique or well defined.

Of course, I am not dismissing the fact that there are diverse abnormalities found in fibromyalgia. For example, certain abnormalities in neurotransmitters have been discovered, but are these the cause or the effect of chronic pain? More recently, my colleague Rick Gracely from the National Institute of Health in Bethesda, Maryland, and his collaborators studied the brains of fibromyalgia patients with fMRI (functional magnetic resonance imaging) and compared them with those of normal people.[21] The researchers found that in patients with fibromyalgia, several areas of their brain were activated by low-grade pressure on their thumbnails, but such pressure failed to produce the same degree of brain activation in the normal subjects. They concluded that the results can be attributed to pathologic sensitivity to pain of fibromyalgia patients at brain levels. On the other hand, many studies show significant psychosocial and environmental issues in patients diagnosed with fibromyalgia.[22] Such studies have led other researchers to attribute the abnormal sensitivity to pain observed in patients with fibromyalgia to psychological factors, which result in switching attention more easily toward "detecting pain."

These and several other research findings, as well as the multiple treatments that fail to produce dramatic changes to the sufferers, attest to the nonuniformity of syndromes that are lumped together as one disorder and the variable influence of biomedical and psychosocial factors. The truth is that recognizing a chronic pain disorder only within its biomedical perspective (as happened in the beginning, when fibromyalgia was first established) and ignoring the psychological and socio-environmental contributors to it, is shortsighted and undoubtedly leads to failed management. Recent studies indicate good response by patients with fibromyalgia to multidisciplinary treatments that employ educational and behavioural-cognitive techniques, together with physical exercises. Such treatments address function and the body-mind interaction, and in my mind, they hold much better promise for the sufferers. When the pendulum swings between the biomedical and the psychological perspective, I suspect the truth is somewhere in between.

Donna came to see me in the mid-1990s at the age of 41. She had been involved in a car accident three years before, an accident that scared her stiff and made her unable to drive since because of intense fear. By the time she came to my clinic, she was complaining of diffuse body pain. The mere touch of my fingertip would make her wince with pain. Lying in bed hurt her flesh. She was terribly depressed and withdrawn, fatigued, in worse pain in the damp cold winter days, and, unable to work, dependent on her family for support. She had been investigated to the hilt with all kinds of X-rays, CAT scans and electrophysiological tests, but no cause of her diffuse pains, fatigue and sleep problems had been found. Donna, as one might suspect, had been diagnosed with fibromyalgia by the time she was referred to me.

Despite her intense tenderness to light finger pressure, she was unable to feel the feathery touch of a makeup brush or the prick of a pinwheel over her skin along the whole left side of her body, including her face, arm, torso and leg. She admitted that her pains were actually much worse on the left side. Further investigations in my unit concluded that she also suffered from depression, which was serious and needed specific treatment. We felt strongly that the loss of sensation in the left side of the body was the result of some change in the way her brain perceived her body. I sent Donna to an intense multidisciplinary chronic pain management program at Chedoke McMaster, then run by Dr. Eldon Tunks. Tunks, a psychiatrist, had founded this program more than

25 years before. Such programs employ intense psychosocial rehabilitation in an in-patient setting over an extended period, four weeks at least. Patients with chronic pain disorders are looked at from both the biomedical and psychosocial perspective, in an effort to empower them and give them skills to manage the pain. They undergo significant physical conditioning coupled with education in pain-coping and pain-blocking techniques. Psychiatrists, psychologists, social workers, physiotherapists, occupational therapists, kinesiologists and others form a team to treat such patients in groups, as well as in individual sessions.

Donna returned to me a year after she finished the program and brought me a pair of golden earrings after her recent trip to her homeland, Italy. She told me with shining eyes that Tunks's program "was the best thing that happened to her" since her accident. For the first time, when she got involved with the Chedoke team, she opened up her heart and mourned openly the loss of her long-time lover who had died from a heart attack two months after the car accident (something she never disclosed to me or my staff). Donna had buried the emotional pain deeply in her heart and had never told anyone anything about this tragic story, until she felt more comfortable during the intense encounters with the Chedoke group. Once she opened up her heart, she was more capable of dealing with the diffuse pain, she formed long-term friendships with other patients and she managed to engage in some part-time courses. Donna's pain did not go away (although it does disappear when she travels to warm Italy). But it is much less intense and she manages it better with the techniques she was taught and with very little medication. Remarkably, the decreased sensation in the left side of her body remains, a permanent mark of the brain's bizarre response to the combined forces of the acute physical trauma of muscle injury during the accident, the fear of almost having been killed and the emotional despair and devastation from the loss of her loved one shortly after the accident. In my mind, the combination of all these co-existing events left a near-permanent imprint in Donna's brain and raised her sensitivity to feel pain on gentle pressure of the finger tip, while her skin on the left side remained insensitive to other pressure stimuli. But, how does one put together such unexplainable body reactions—too little and too much sensitivity at the same time?

Donna's decreased sensation in half of her body puzzled me. She was similar to so many others who were referred to my clinic bearing the diagnosis of fibromyalgia. A hypothesis formed gradually in my mind: We know that our bodies send all kinds of signals to our brains every minute. Whispering signals of minor discomfort, which, despite the fact that we do not feel consciously through the night as we sleep, warn the body enough to make us change positions and avoid constant pressure on the same side for many hours. Louder signals reach our consciousness and make us take off our narrow shoes when we feel a blister forming. Finally, when a rock crashes on our foot, the pain "screams" to make us not only pull the foot away, but also to feel the hurt intensely. As our attention, emotions and previous experiences come in, the signals and the voices of pain may be suppressed as unconscious whispers, or they may become deafening screams. Remember our earlier discussion of how the body has some kind of attentional filter that labels what is important and what is unimportant for the brain to consider? In my view, Donna's filter got damaged by events—the combined effect of physical and emotional trauma coupled with her major loss of her partner. When I contemplate this, all I can do is marvel. The thought that something has happened to change her brain's sensitivity and make her feel things much more (manifested by her flesh pain), and at the same time also much less (the loss of her skin's sensation) is a daring one—it may seem obvious after her story has been told, but in the typical biomedical model of disease, it is unorthodox. While this concept seemed far-fetched to me some years ago, it is not any more, as research now supports this concept of altered brain activity in fibromyalgia and other unexplainable persistent pains.

In many such cases, what seems to be increased sensitivity toward feeling pain may relate to the switching of attention toward internal painful stimuli. My team and I go further. We question the possibility that this altered brain activity may be the result of interplay of emotional and personality factors together with some physical trauma, which in turn switches the focus of attention to picking up pain signals more easily,[23] a state that some researchers label as "hypervigilance." In those cases, teaming up the patient with a group of trained health care workers (doctors, psychologists, exercise and other therapists, social workers and so on) seems to be a solid approach. The patient has to be a part of the team.

Seven

INTERNAL ORGANS AND INJURED NERVES

Christina was 26 when she came to me, with a decade of pain literally under her belt. She had a history of chronic pelvic pain that had begun when she started menstruating at the age of 14. In the beginning, her pain would come only with her periods, but by 19 it became constant. At 21 she had a laparoscopy—her gynecologist inserted a small tube through her navel to examine her inner organs. Small patches of endometriosis were found. Endometriosis is a condition in which parts of the lining of the uterus migrate into the abdominal cavity and produce inflammation and scar tissue. After the procedure, Christina was placed on medication, since the doctors suspected that her endometriosis had something to do with her pain. But the drugs did not help and she had another laparoscopy a year later to clean the scar tissue; this did not help either. Within a year, she was hooked on opioids and had to be admitted to a detoxification centre.

I often ask patients to rate their pain on a scale of 0 to 10, with 10 being the worst pain. Christina rated hers a 7. But when I examined her in my in-patient unit, I couldn't find anything wrong with her, except perhaps some vague tenderness across her whole abdominal wall. We put Christina through a round of tests, as we do for all patients whose symptoms aren't easily analyzed. She saw several of our consultants, including the psychiatrist and the psychologist on my team. During some of the tests we performed, including the administration of different types of medications intravenously, we noticed something unusual: Christina had lost all her pains. No matter how hard I poked, no matter how hard she pushed her tummy and searched, there was no sign of the discomfort that had sent her to us in the first place. So, if the pain was not coming from within her own body, where was it coming from?

Christina's personal history was important to her diagnosis. She came from a strict Italian family. She fell in love in her mid-teens with a boy who wrote poetry. They were close, but she resisted his sexual advances for many months. Because she was a devout Catholic, she was "saving herself" for marriage. Finally, though, she gave in to her boyfriend's pressure, only to have him dump her within a month.

Christina was devastated. Soon after, she met an older man and started having sex with him daily, and a year later she moved in with him. It was then that her intermittent pain turned serious and more or less constant. Christina confessed that her lover was involved in sado-masochistic activities and got her involved too, not only at home but also at a special club. She ended up working there. Her role with customers was that of the "slave," or the submissive partner. Christina became terribly depressed and started using large doses of Percocet again (an opioid from the morphine family). She would consume up to 20 tablets per day, a few of them prescribed by her doctor, most of them bought on the street. She attempted to quit taking these narcotics "cold turkey" and went through a cruel, vicious withdrawal—sweating, palpitations and abdominal pains. Then she broke up with her lover and for several months her pain subsided remarkably, without any medication. But when she got into trouble in her workplace, her pains started mounting again.

In the middle of all this, she met a customer at the club, a younger man who seemed to have fallen in love with her, and Christina was hopeful that this relationship could work. All of this—her puritanical background, her sorrow from being dumped, her adventures in the demimonde, her newfound hope—was of clinical interest to us, in terms of helping us understand the psychological roots of Christina's pain.

Marina, another patient, turned out to be one of my most complicated and unfortunate cases. She was the executive assistant for a member of Parliament, 28 years old, happily married and expecting her second child. Life was really going well for her. But when her water broke, what seemed to be a normally progressing labour ended up a major disaster. The baby was not coming out the right way, and vacuum suction had to be used. Unfortunately, too much suction was applied and it tore Marina's bladder and vagina, creating a fistula—an unhealthy connection—between these two viscera. The doctors attempted to repair the fistula by using a graft—a piece of tissue from Marina's labia (the outer lips of her vagina). Marina was left with numerous problems, including severe pain and bladder incontinence. She was sent to a particular specialist, who applied a sacral nerve stimulator—an electrical device to power the opening of her bladder, to help her hold her urine—but this failed. Marina was also given many pain medications, with little relief. By the time she came to see me, she was extremely depressed—who wouldn't be? She had put on a fair amount of weight, she could not sleep, the medications made her vomit all the time and she hurt constantly.

Marina actually had more than one pain. She described a sharp steady one in her lower tummy, a knife-like pain close to her vagina (she was told that this was coming from bladder spasms), and finally severe burning in her labia, from the site of the graft. When I first read her history, it was alarming enough. When I saw her, I could not contain my horror.

Marina could not sit and paced the room. Even as we talked, tears ran down her face. When I examined her, apart from severe tenderness when my fingers tried to feel her abdomen, she had some surprising changes in her skin sensation.

I have several ways to test the feeling of the skin, as different types of sensation are transmitted by different types of nerve fibres all the way to the brain. The large A-beta fibres carry the touch of a feathery little brush, while the small fibres (primarily C fibres) carry the sensation of sharpness from the pointy spokes of a pinwheel over the skin. When I did these tests on Marina's abdomen, she was surprisingly sensitive to the touch of my brush and the pinwheel over a large area, from her breasts to midway down her thighs. While I knew already that she had significant damage in several inner organs, the finding of diffuse and abnormal skin sensitivity added another piece to her pain puzzle. The damage was much beyond the nociceptors of the vagina and bladder wall: it had affected several of the nerves that supply these viscera. In other words, she had not only visceral somatic pain but also neuropathic pain.

Furthermore, the changes in her nervous system had progressed to "central sensitization" (a concept discussed in Chapter five). This results from the constant barrage of abnormally firing injured nerves, sensitizing certain cells in the spinal cord and making them respond intensely to stimuli coming from the body. Central sensitization is not only responsible for adding to the pain but also for producing profound changes in the sensation of the skin. Marina's skin bore all the marks of this phenomenon, but to make sure, I administered a drug called sodium amytal, which is applied intravenously. When the drug entered her vein, the pain of touch (which is called allodynia when normally non-painful stimuli invoke pain) diminished quite a bit, while Marina's sensitivity to pinpricks decreased only slightly. This response to sodium amytal confirmed my suspicion of central sensitization.[1]

Marina had come from another province to see us, and we sent her back to her doctors with a number of suggestions. We felt that her depression was as severe as the damage to her body, and that both needed equal attention. A year and a half later Marina came back to see me. She had gone through megadoses of neuropathic medications and morphine-like drugs with not much help until her psychiatrist vigorously attacked her depression with a combination of antidepressants and counselling. This worked better. Marina finally managed to accept that she had suffered physical damage that was permanent and severe and that she was never going to be the way she was before. Once she accepted her limitations, she was able to ask herself, "How do I make the best of what I have?"

With this insight, plus support from her family and her doctors, the antidepressant medications started working. When I saw her, all the signs of severe visceral and neuropathic pain were still there, and Marina was still taking drugs for the pain. But for the first time, she had a smile on her beautiful face. I praised the strength of her mind and soul. "Marina," I said, "you must know by now it is not our medications alone that make so much of a difference. The big difference comes from within you. We as doctors try to help you. But if you were not going to help yourself first, everything we know and do would not work." When I had first met Marina, I had told her as she was leaving my office in despair: "Never lose your smile before I do, and I never do." This time we both had a smile.

Christina had chronic pain that started with her periods and evolved to chronic, unremitting pelvic pain, influenced mainly by stress and emotional turmoil. Marina sustained serious internal damage and ended up with both visceral nociceptive pain and neuropathic pain, both of which were made worse by her depression. Both of these women's pains fell into the category of chronic pelvic pain—a problem of considerable dimensions. A friend of mine, Dr. Ursula Wesselman, an expert in this type of pain in the United States, reviewed results from several studies.[2] She found that chronic pelvic pain accounts for 40 per cent of all laparoscopies and 12 to 16 per cent of hysterectomies done yearly in the United States. This works out to 80,000 surgeries per year in the United States alone. Altogether, it is estimated that 30 to 50 per cent of the 45 million women in the U.S. who are in their childbearing years suffer from painful periods or cyclic pain. Furthermore, about 15 per cent of the women with chronic pelvic pain lose time from work and 45 per cent report reduced productivity. Medical costs for outpatient visits for chronic pelvic pain in the U.S. are U.S.$881.5 million per year; the cost to women in terms of suffering, disability, relationship problems, loss of jobs and frustration after ineffective medical procedures cannot be as easily calculated. Unfortunately, as fascinating as it is to researchers, pelvic pain is difficult to understand and manage because more than one-third of the women who suffer from it do not have obvious pathology. It's not easy for the doctor to say what is wrong.

One challenge that doctors face is that chronic pelvic pain is not necessarily of gynecological origin alone. The bladder, the ureters (tubes connecting the kidneys to the bladder), parts of the gut, and even pain from muscles and joints or neurological problems may give rise to pain felt in the pelvis and lower abdomen. As my own experience with Christina and Marina exemplifies, there can be a significant relationship between pelvic pain and psychological factors.

A review of the scientific literature in this field backs this up.[3] For example, 28 per cent of women with pelvic pain suffer from depression, compared with only 3 per cent of women who visit gynecologists for reasons other than pelvic pain. How much of the pain causes the depression and how much of the depression causes the pain?

Research further shows that a history of childhood sexual abuse is higher among patients with chronic pelvic pain (58 per cent) compared with gynecological patients without pain or even patients with other kinds of pain (30 per cent).[4] The complex nature of chronic pelvic pain makes medical assessment by the doctor a complicated matter—you have to be extremely thorough before drawing up a comprehensive treatment plan. Treating women through non-surgical approaches should always be tried first. Some of the greatest successes in treating chronic pelvic pain seem to come when patients get involved in multidisciplinary pain programs, in which specialist doctors and other health care professionals work together to address pain from both the physical and the psychological perspectives.

The pain described above is an example of one kind of visceral pain, that coming from the pelvic viscera. But similar pains may come from viscera outside the pelvis, such as the heart, the esophagus (our food pipe), the stomach, the bowels or the gall bladder. If you have ever felt a horrible chest pain and thought immediately that this is what a heart attack must feel like, you'll have an idea of what one of my patients, Martin experienced.

Martin, who was tall, blonde and muscular, had immigrated to Canada from the Netherlands in his mid-30s; he was 48 when I admitted him to my in-patient unit. An emergency nurse, he had practised at home and had earned a degree in a Canadian college. He had been referred to me after complaining of serious chest pain. His cardiologist had investigated him thoroughly and was convinced that whatever was wrong with Martin was not coming from an ailing heart. His electrocardiogram (ECG) showed few abnormalities. All kinds of other heart tests had failed to show much either. The mystery was solved when I offered Martin an admission to my in-patient unit. I happened to stay late one night to finish work that was piling on my desk, when I was called onto the ward. Martin was lying in bed, short of breath, clutching his chest and drenched in sweat.

He pointed to his heart. Even to an untrained eye, let alone my trained one, he looked as if he was having a heart attack. However, the ECG was no different than before and his pain would not go away despite the several nitroglycerin tablets that Martin had put under his tongue (nitroglycerin is used by heart patients to dilate the coronary arteries that bring blood to the heart muscle). So I made a quick decision. Instead of treating Martin's heart, I decided to treat what I perceived was high anxiety.

I gave Martin some quick-acting medication from the same family as valium. He placed the tablet under his tongue. It was absorbed quickly, directly into the bloodstream. This settled Martin's anxiety enough to enable him to answer more questions. It seemed that this pain spell followed a fairly heavy meal; Martin, like so many people, disliked the hospital food and ordered in something else. When I learned of his spicy dinner, I prescribed some heavy antacids, which indeed settled Martin's chest pain. The next morning I lined up Martin for more investigations. This time I targeted his stomach and esophagus instead of his heart. I was right. Martin had "non-cardiac chest pain" disguised as angina, due to problems with his esophagus.

Chest pain is frightening. It comes second after abdominal pain as the most frequent cause for emergency visits to the doctor. Pain coming from the heart (cardiac pain) is called angina. Patients describe it as heaviness, tightness or squeezing, usually behind the breastbone. Sometimes the pain is felt in the upper part of the abdomen and may be referred to the left arm, jaw and neck or teeth. In some people, the discomfort may be experienced only in these areas and not the chest at all. The pain seems to be most often provoked by strenuous activity. Its cause is usually ischemia of the heart muscle, which happens when the coronary arteries are clogged. In such situations, there is not enough blood to bring oxygen to the heart muscle during physical activity. Other times, angina may occur when the coronary arteries go into spasm. Sometimes, however, some of these blood-starving episodes or even true heart attacks fail to create pain, so we have what we call "silent ischemia." The truth is that chest pains do not come only from the heart. About 20 per cent of the patients who complain of chest pain and undergo cardiac catheterization are found to have normal coronary arteries.[5]

Chest pains may arise outside the heart, from the esophagus, the lungs, from inflammation or trauma of the chest wall (ribs and muscles) or even as part of anxiety attacks. Clinical studies suggest that 10 to 30 per cent of patients with suspected angina may actually be suffering from esophageal chest pain.[6]

Some patients who experience chest pain but have normal coronary arteries may simply have an increased sensitivity of the heart to pain.[7] And in many, more than one factor seems to be present. In a study of such patients with chest pain but normal coronary arteries, some ischemia showed up in the ECGs in only 22 per cent; 41 per cent had problems with the motility of their esophagus (the ability of the esophagus's muscular layer to propel food); 63 per cent had co-existent psychiatric disorders, particularly panic attacks; and 87 per cent had increased cardiac sensitivity to painful stimuli. In other words, there was often more than one reason for these pains, but only a small part of the pain was coming from problems of true ischemia within the coronary arteries. This same study showed that 50 per cent of these patients responded quite well to a drug called imipramine, which is a type of tricyclic antidepressant. Not only did their moods improve, but also the sensitivity of the heart to painful stimuli (at least as tested in the laboratory) was much reduced.

Non-cardiac chest pain does not come cheap.[8] It was estimated that the cost of such pains in 1995 in the U.S. alone exceeded $1 billion. Even when patients are assured that they do not have heart disease, as many as 50 per cent continue having debilitating symptoms and suffer considerable social dysfunction.

The patients described so far suffer from different forms of visceral nociceptive pains, sometimes mixed with other forms of pain (neuropathic and somatic nociceptive). Anxiety and depression can make matters more puzzling, as they can seriously affect the degree and intensity of pain. Pain and individual responses to treatment are complex and varied, which is why it is so important for doctors to look at all the possible components of a patient's suffering.

Visceral nociceptive pains are difficult to understand and treat. Neuropathic pains are even worse. Albert, a 67-year-old retired real estate agent, was sent to me by his family physician. His problem started four years earlier when he suffered a stroke. During a stroke, a part of the brain gets damaged and literally dies because a blood clot in an artery cuts its blood supply or, to the contrary, because a blood vessel bursts (often because of high blood pressure). In Albert's case, the stroke damaged the right side of his brain. Since the left brain controls the right side of the body and vice versa, it was Albert's left arm and leg that were paralyzed. By the time he came to see me, his left side was stiff and weak, his fingers were curled up and he could hardly stand without holding onto someone. He complained bitterly about pain in his arm and leg in the affected side, which appeared almost the same day of his stroke. Albert described it as constant, stabbing, pounding, aching and cramping. Any attempt to move his limbs, emotional stress or cold and damp weather would make the pain worse. Albert rated his pain as 6 out of 10. When I examined him, his face, arm, leg and even his chest, belly and back on the left side were extremely sensitive to the feathery touch of my light makeup brush and the sharp teeth of my pinwheel.

Sydney, on the other hand, had a serious car accident in 1987, at the age of 23. Young and daring, with too much testosterone in his body and a mix of booze and pot in his brain, he drove too fast. When they collected him from the ditch on a board, Sydney knew something terrible had happened. He could not move or feel his arms and legs. He had crushed his neck. He actually had a fracture of the fifth cervical vertebra with damage of the spinal cord at this level, and he became a quadriplegic. Within a year of the injury, he recovered some strength in his upper arms. Pains in his belly, back and right leg appeared slowly within this first year. He described them as cramping, burning, aching and shooting, rated them as 7 out of 10 and said that the bellyache was worse every time he had a bladder infection. When I examined him, Sydney perceived the touch of the brush and the pricking of the pinwheel only down to his collar bone. Below that, he had no feeling at all, and he could not even wiggle his toes.

Gordana was 21 years old and three months pregnant when she got a "bad flu." Sniffles, sneezing, headaches, high fever and aching muscles lasted for several days and she still felt lousy for weeks. By the end of the fourth month of her pregnancy, she started feeling a severe burning pain in her rectum and vagina, and her balance was really off. She would wobble and walk like a duck. The pain did not get better when her baby daughter was born. Gordana would spend a whole day with an ice pack between her legs to control the burning. She was in so much pain that she could not sit, could not take care of the baby and could not concentrate. Several tests were done to figure out the origin of this bizarre and debilitating pain. Her doctors concluded that she had suffered "transverse myelitis," an inflammation of the spinal cord, believed to be a reaction to her bad flu. In my office, a year and a half later, Gordana seemed in great distress. She walked with an unstable, wobbly gait, her legs were stiff and they shook— the medical term for the combination of stiffness, weakness and shakes is "spacticity." When I tested her reflexes, her tendon jerks were abnormally hyper-active. The feathery touch of my little brush over her inner thighs and her private parts bothered her profoundly.

While the diagnosis of neuropathic pain was made rather easily and quickly in the patients I just discussed, for others it takes many years to find out the source of pain. Twelve years before he visited my office, Stephen, 50, started complaining badly about pain in both shoulders and his upper back. Since the doctors could not find the origin of his pain, he was labelled as having "fibromyalgia." Years later, however, his right shoulder started showing signs of serious damage. Then the doctors changed their mind about fibromyalgia and diagnosed Stephen with severe osteoarthritis. It was so bad that he had surgery to put in an artificial joint to his right shoulder. Unfortunately, although his shoulder movements improved, his pain became more serious and burning. It was not until 1993, almost eight years after the onset of his pain, that the doctors, puzzled by the persistence of the pain, decided to investigate his brain and spinal cord. At that time, an MRI showed that Stephen was born with an anomaly of his lower brain, called Chiari malformation. This abnormality is very often associated with "syringomyelia"—in which a cavity called a syrinx is formed within the spinal cord. Most times these cavities occur because of abnormal drainage of the cerebrospinal fluid that circulates between the brain and the spinal cord, as it happens with Chiari malformation. In other instances, syringomyelic cavities are the result of scarring within the spinal cord, for example after a spinal cord injury like the one Sydney had suffered in his car accident. In syringomyelia, the damage of nervous tissue may lead to destruc-tion of joints, which could explain the problem with Stephen's shoulder. Stephen ended up having several surgeries to release the pressure from his lower brain and empty the excess fluid from his syrinx. By the time he came to see me, he had pains all over his body—in his shoulders, flanks, right leg, both wrists and behind his left eye, where he felt a stabbing pain, in addition to the nearly constant headaches at the back of his head. He was very depressed. This once sturdy man had many patches of distorted sensation throughout his body.

In some areas he could not feel my feathery brush or my pinwheel, while in other areas even the touch of a Kleenex was unbearable.

All the patients I described had a common problem. They suffered from what we call "central neuropathic pain." That is a handy descriptive term for neuropathic pains caused by damage to the central nervous system (the brain and the spinal cord). In Albert's case, it was "central post-stroke pain," after brain damage. Sydney, Stephen and Gordana suffered from pain resulting from damage of the spinal cord.

It is estimated that about 8 per cent of all patients with stroke will end up with some kind of post-stroke pain syndrome.[9] For roughly a third of those unlucky patients who develop this problem, the pain will appear almost immediately after the stroke; for about half, it will show up anywhere from a few days to a year later; but for the remainder of the pain sufferers it can take as long as two years for it to appear. In the case of spinal cord damage, pain will develop in up to 94 per cent of patients from within days to many months. Trauma like the one suffered by Sydney is the most common cause. Three-fourths of the patients who suffer this injury are males. Spinal cord injury may generate all kinds of pains—for example, burning coming from the damaged spinal cord itself, or the nerve roots at the level of the lesion, bladder and "gut" aches, and pains in the muscles and bones at the point where the injury occurred or above.

Patients with brain or spinal cord damage suffer from more than one pain, each of which may be of different duration, quality and intensity. Some pains are constant, some others come and go abruptly in spells and others are felt when pressure, touch or prick is applied to the painful area. Neuropathic pains are generally difficult to treat. Usually, my first line of attack involves what we call neuropathic medications—tricyclic antidepressants and/or anticonvulsants. The latter are drugs used against epilepsy; they also also stabilize irritable nerve membranes. Patients with neuropathic pain often need opioids such as morphine, too. Sometimes treatment includes implanting electrodes on the spinal cord or even into the brain. The latter method is obviously a rather aggressive intervention and is therefore reserved for the most intractable cases. In rare cases, to eliminate abnormal signals, neurosurgeons will actually damage or cut a part of the spinal cord or the brain.

Albert was prescribed small doses of anticonvulsants and painkillers, to be taken around the clock. He did not do well with these medications while he was alone at home and had plenty of time to kill. But he did much better when his wife put him in a special day hospital program, where his mind was kept busy constantly. Sydney and Stephen needed a fair amount of morphine on top of neuropathic medications. Both had only moderate relief and they were constantly fighting depression.

Their results disappointed me—when one works at a pain clinic, one hopes the patients' pain will get better. Gordana, though, was a miracle. I started her on small doses of the antidepressant amitriptyline. Six weeks later I did not recognize her. The distraught, unkempt and depressed young lady who had been unable to sit or hold her baby showed up looking terrific, wearing a flowery dress, high heels, makeup and with her long hair in a ponytail. Her gait was still a little wobbly, but the high heels could be blamed for that more than her condition. Her makeup, too, was rather flamboyant, but who really cared? She was accompanied by her husband, whose adoring eyes, fixed on her huge smile, were more than enough for me. She could not stop telling me how much better she felt. At times, her pains still return with a vengeance. But as we got to know her at our clinic, we realized that whenever she experiences a minor flare-up, she goes into panic. When that happens, we temporarily add to her medication a minor anti-anxiety drug or switch in an additional simple analgesic. In her case we felt it is important to treat both the pain itself and the anxiety that surrounds the pain.

Unfortunately, neuropathic pains are not well understood either by patients or many doctors. Pain is a significant problem in some commonly occurring diseases like multiple sclerosis (MS) and Parkinson's disease. It is only in the last 10 to 15 years that physicians have come to realize that up to two-thirds of people with multiple sclerosis suffer pain.[10] MS attacks the central nervous system and produces weakness, stiffness, tremors and at times paralysis. MS-related pains can be central neuropathic (with burning affecting the legs), peripheral neuropathic (affecting otherwise unafflicted parts of the body due to pinched nerves in the legs and arms) or even nociceptive musculoskeletal—aching over muscles and bones.

As with MS, it is only over the past 10 years or so that we have come to understand the nature of pains in patients with Parkinson's disease. Parkinson's is a degenerative disease that affects certain structures in the brain called basal ganglia, responsible for the smooth co-ordination of our movements. This disease has been given extensive publicity lately, because of Muhammad Ali, who has it, and because of the actor Michael J. Fox, who left the hit TV series *Spin City* after doctors determined that his suffering from jerks, tremors, rigidity and unwanted movements meant that he had Parkinson's. We owe a lot of thanks to them for their courage in confronting their disease and thereby demystifying Parkinson's and helping to raise money for research leading to better treatments. Remarkably, though, even now relatively few physicians seem to know that pain occurs in between 10 and 30 per cent of all patients with Parkinson's.[11] These pains are mostly intermittent, diffuse and poorly localized, affecting the head, face, neck, torso and limbs. Until recently, it was thought that most of these pains were related to the effect or lack of effect of anti-Parkinson's medications. Today we know that the basal ganglia play a role in pain perception and modulation, and that many of these pains are central pains, irrespective of the effect of Parkinson's drugs.

Mark had a particularly difficult case of Parkinson's disease with severe pain. He was 56 when I saw him some years ago. He was diagnosed with Parkinson's at 48; he had been a police officer but had to retire soon after the diagnosis was made. Mark's disease was hard to treat. He agreed to participate in an experimental treatment called glial derived neurotrophic factor, which involved injections of a special substance inside his brain. Unfortunately, after the treatment he got no better; in fact he got worse, and for this reason his neurologist referred him to me. By the time I saw him, he was complaining bitterly of severe cramps in his legs, burning in his feet and painful spasms in his left leg. On examination I found that his left foot was hypersensitive to touch and pinprick and would go into extension, like a ballet dancer's pointed foot, from time to time. In addition, his other limbs were stiff.

I suspected that Mark was suffering from not just one affliction but a combination of pains and pain mechanisms: he probably had a small-fibre neuropathy to account for his burning foot pain plus a central neuropathic type of pain associated with Parkinson's disease. I thought the neuropathy may have been an unexpected complication of the experimental treatment he had received. Mark responded well to a special pain medication called a Duragesic patch.

The patch, which can be placed over the limbs or elsewhere on the body, delivers an opioid called fentanyl (synthesized from morphine) at a steady rate through the skin. But the pain relief lasted only one year. As the tremors and rigidity progressed, though, Mark's treatment got more complicated. He ended up having two deep brain stimulators surgically inserted directly into his brain. A deep brain stimulator consists basically of an electrical generator, which delivers pulses by means of electrodes placed on the surface of a specific region of the brain that is thought to be causing the pain. The source of power to the generator is supplied by an implanted battery or by an external radio transmitter.

The stimulators worked very well for a period of time. Mark experienced dramatic improvement in both the Parkinson's symptoms and his leg pains, to the point that he did not need analgesics. But a year and a half after the stimulators were inserted, the burning pain started returning to both legs. When Mark revisited me in 2001, his pains were intermittent but the left foot was permanently twisted. By this time, feeling that both this foot position (called dystonic foot posturing) and the intermittent pain episodes were of central origin, I decided to try something else. I added an anti-epileptic medication, to cut down on abnormally firing cells in his central nervous system. Mark has done fairly well since with the combination of deep brain stimulation, anti-Parkinson's drugs, analgesic and neuropathic medications.

Neuropathic pains are a large family, and central neuropathic pains are only part of this family. There are numerous other pains that affect the peripheral part of the nervous system, the nerves and nerve roots, called peripheral neuropathic pains.

Many people have heard of the phenomenon of "ghost pain," or phantom limb pain, which is the strange sensation experienced by a person who has lost a hand, a foot, an arm or a leg. In different studies, between half and nearly three-quarters (53 to 72 per cent) of patients who lose a limb because of poor blood supply or trauma will continue to feel this ghost pain in the limb that is no longer there.[12] The pain lasts for many years or indefinitely. Studies in both monkeys and humans have helped us understand that when the body's shape gets altered, for example, by loss of a limb, the brain is "re-organized." In phantom limb pain, both changes in the peripheral and the central nervous system contribute to the generation of pain. Changes in the local nerves of the stump contribute to a constant barrage of abnormal discharges from these nerves, which feed into the already abnormal brain map. People experience phantom limb pain not only after losing a leg or arm but also after the loss of a breast to cancer, or even the loss of a penis or rectum. These extreme losses happen when cancer invades those areas and the surgeon has no other options but to remove them to halt the progression of the tumours. Phantom limb pain is a mixed form of neuropathic pain, with abnormal discharges from both the nerves of the stump, as well as the spinal cord and the brain.

Esther was 69 when she came to see me. She woke up one morning a year earlier with burning pain on her left side underneath her breast. Two days later she discovered blisters in the area where she felt the pain. The blisters crusted and dried but the pain continued. Esther had a bout of acute shingles. The disease is caused by the varicella zoster virus (VZV), which typically we get as children in the form of chicken pox. After the chicken pox is over, the virus lies dormant in the dorsal root ganglia, the lumps of tissue that contain the cells of the peripheral nerves just outside the spinal cord. Shingles is caused by the activation of the sleeping virus as we get older, or in patients whose immune system is weak (for example those with AIDS or cancer). Shingles affects approximately 131 persons per 100,000 people every year, and our risk increases substantially as we get older. Most patients with a bout of shingles and acute pain will not develop chronic pain (post-herpetic neuralgia). When the pain of shingles persists after three months, 12 per cent of sufferers will still hurt for at least a year.[13] However, post-herpetic neuralgia is much more frequent in people older than 65. This is exactly what Esther had developed. When I examined her, she had patches of thin, scarred skin on her left side. In some of these spots she could not tolerate even the touch of her clothes, while in other spots she did not know when I pressed my finger against her. She had intermittent stabs of knife-like pain amid a background of constant throbbing and burning.

Shingles can be treated by pills or by creams, depending on the individual, the degree of discomfort and the intensity of the post-herpetic neuralgia.[14] Some people respond well to tricyclic antidepressants—amitriptyline is the prototypical drug. Tricyclic antidepressants work by inhibiting the elimination of some special neurotransmitters (serotonine and noradrenaline), which are involved in pain transmission. They also suppress abnormal firing in the central nervous system. Studies show that tricyclic antidepressants will provide considerable relief in about 50 per cent of shingles cases. Other pills that can help include opioid medications for analgesia and anti-epileptic medications.

In terms of creams, or what doctors call local treatments, capsaicin cream (known commercially as Zostrix) is the only topical drug approved in the United States and Canada for post-herpetic neuralgia. Capsaicin is the extract of red hot chili peppers. It is the stuff that sets you on fire when you eat spicy food. It is also in the pepper spray used by the police. Capsaicin works by emptying the terminal nerve endings of the small pain fibres from a particular neurotransmitter called substance P. Once substance P is depleted from the nerve terminals, the nerve fibres stop conveying pain signals. Unfortunately, almost one-third of the patients who try capsaicin abandon it. In cream form, capsaicin creates an intense burning sensation at the beginning of the treatment, and many people simply can't stand it. Another topical treatment that some people use contains a local freezing agent (lidocaine); it can be applied either as a cream or on a patch stuck to the skin. Unfortunately, non-medicinal treatments like acupuncture and transcutaneous electrical nerve stimulation (TENS) don't seem to be effective in post-herpetic neuralgia. Similarly, nerve blocks (injections into nerve tissues such as the stellate ganglion by the side of the neck, over the nerves of the chest wall or into the spine) seem to work for only a few patients. Esther was lucky. She responded well to small doses of desipramine, a drug similar to amitriptyline, and went on her merry way after a few visits to my clinic.

Marcel had a different problem. At the age of 45 he started suffering spells of excruciating pain on his face. He would experience brief stabbing or shock-like episodes of immense intensity across his left cheek and forehead. The pain spells would come on their own, or would be provoked by chewing food or by a mere breeze over his face. This rare condition is called trigeminal neuralgia, as the outbursts of pain specifically involve the trigeminal nerve, one of the nerves that supply the skin of the face. This nerve has three branches. In Marcel's case, the branches of his forehead and cheek were responsible for the episodes of unbearable pain. Marcel was lucky, as he responded extremely well to an anti-epileptic drug, carbamazepine (commercially known as Tegretol).

Esther's and Marcel's experiences are examples of peripheral neuropathic pain. But the list of damaged nerves does not end there. Nerve damage is the result of disease, traumas and surgeries, or the side effect of certain drug treatments. Peripheral neuropathic pains are not rare. Patients with diabetes often develop diabetic neuropathy, and in some cases this is painful. Such patients complain of numbness and aching, stabbing or burning pain, primarily in their feet and lower legs. About one in four women who have had breast surgery still complain of pain 12 months after the operation (very frequently resulting from damage of local nerves). And, after a thoracotomy (opening of the chest cavity to correct an abdominal hernia or to perform lung surgery), 14 per cent of the patients continue to complain of pain after a year, and often indefinitely. This pain also comes from damage to local nerves.

Back in 1989, my team and I reported to *Heart and Lung*, a journal for cardiologists and cardiovascular surgeons, about a bizarre group of patients who would come to see me after cardiac bypass surgery. These patients complained of severe ongoing burning pain and could not tolerate contact from their clothes, or from running water over their chest or even from a slight breeze. Their intolerance to touch is what I described as "allodynia" earlier, in Marina's case. Alarmed by the appearance of such an unusual group, we investigated the origin of their pain. We concluded that during surgery, the surgeons had damaged the nerves of the chest wall (called intercostal nerves) in an effort to fetch a small artery called the internal mammary or thoracic artery. This artery would serve as a graft to help replace one of the diseased coronary arteries that supply the heart muscle with blood. Since my group was the first in the world to describe such an entity, we had the privilege of naming it, and we called it internal mammary artery syndrome.[15] Eleven years later, we published another study showing that nearly three-quarters of all patients who undergo cardiac bypass surgery that involves this type of graft end up with damaged intercostal nerves. Fifteen per cent of those with nerve damage continue to have significant pain two and a half years or more after the surgery.[16]

Let's think about these numbers for a moment. My own hospital performs more than 1600 such surgeries a year, which means that more than 1000 patients will sustain nerve damage on their chest walls, and about 150 of these will continue to endure significant pain for years. Every year, more than 6500 cardiac bypass surgeries are performed in the province of Ontario and more than 16,000 in the state of New York. This means that hundreds of heart patients will continue to suffer with chronic chest pain, which more often than not they will attribute to continuous heart problems. They may believe that their heart operation "didn't work" or they may worry, as do their physicians, who in most cases have never heard about this syndrome. Such patients undergo all kinds of heart tests again and again at a significant cost to the health care system. However, the internal mammary artery syndrome is a neuropathic problem and may improve with the use of classic neuropathic medications such as tricyclic anti-depressants and anti-epileptics. Other times, though, patients resort to creating ingenious ways to avoid the unbearable contact with their clothes, so they can go to their job properly dressed.

George actually wore a homemade wooden frame under his shirt, to avoid having his clothes come in contact with his skin. He was a history professor and was sent to me by his cardiologist to figure out why he could not tolerate the touch of his shirt on his skin after his heart bypass surgery. When I diagnosed him with internal mammary artery syndrome, George was somewhat relieved that this pain was not coming from his heart. Nevertheless, he needed to return to teaching ("good for his mind," he said, and I could not agree more). So, ingeniously, he created a wooden frame to go over his neck. He stopped using the frame about two years after the surgery, when the touch pain became much less intense.

Another serious neuropathic syndrome, causalgia, is one we encountered earlier in this book, in Edward's case. The name causalgia is derived from the Greek words *causos* ("burning") and *algos* ("pain"). Causalgia occurs after an injury to a large nerve and causes nearly identical symptoms and signs with another syndrome, reflex sympathetic dystrophy (RSD). Both entities are known now under an all-encompassing umbrella name, complex regional pain syndromes. Causalgia happens when a large nerve gets cut or crushed, but RSD can start from a rather trivial injury like a muscle or joint sprain, or a more serious injury like a broken bone. Either way, the limb may get very painful, swollen, hot and then cold, discoloured and stiff, while the nails get brittle and the hair coarse. The unfortunate patient often is unable to tolerate the touch of a feather over the skin, and the simplest movements cause ripples of pain.

A while ago, scientists started realizing that although the trauma involves just a limb, both the peripheral and central nervous systems are affected.

An example of RSD is a case I encountered in the early 1980s. I got a call from a children's rehabilitation hospital, asking me to admit a 17-year-old girl to my unit. They said they did not know what exactly was wrong with her, but she could not put her right leg on the ground. Her symptoms started after an insignificant ankle sprain. Jenny was brought to my office on a stretcher. Her right leg was skinnier than the left, cold and purple. She had constant pain, she said, often accompanied by acute pains shooting up her leg. She could not tolerate even the touch of the bedsheets. My diagnosis was RSD. I asked the anaesthetists to use a type of nerve block (called a sympathetic block) in Jenny's back in an effort to inhibit part of the nervous system that I felt was malfunctioning. The anaesthetist carefully put a needle into her back to deliver a small quantity of local freezing agent to the sympathetic nerves innervating the leg. The blocks gave her only short-lived relief. When everything failed (medications, nerve blocks, physiotherapy), I went to the neurosurgeons and asked them to give Jenny a trial of spinal cord stimulation (SCS).

A spinal stimulator involves planting a set of wires (electrodes) on the surface of the spinal cord, close to the region that generates the pain. This method of pain control was first used in 1967 in the United States. Over the last 10 years SCS has gained increasing acceptance as a treatment for different types of neuropathic pain. SCS consists basically of an electrical generator that delivers pulses by means of electrodes placed on the surface of a specific region of the spinal cord that is causing the pain. The leads, containing sets of electrodes, can be implanted by a small open surgery or through the skin. The power is supplied by an implanted battery or by an external transmitter. At the time of her treatment, Jenny had to carry a small device that looked like a pager, hooked on her belt, to activate the stimulator. Nowadays, modern devices are completely inside the body. Better designs for these different components have made SCS an easier form of treatment today. Even before the permanent device is implanted, temporary placement of the electrodes over the surface of the spinal cord allows a simple trial to select suitable patients: the electrodes are simply threaded through the skin, with the help of a large needle, to the surface of the spinal cord. SCS is now used for the treatment of a wide variety of problems, including ischemic disease of the legs, angina, causalgia and RSD, failed back syndrome and diabetic neuropathy. Today, it is estimated that 14,000 stimulators are implanted worldwide each year.[17] However, 15 years ago when I was working with Jenny, the spinal stimulators were considered experimental.

The neurosurgeons I called about Jenny turned me down. "She is too young and too emotional, so she will fail," they said. Besides, since the stimulator was not covered by the provincial health care system, they did not want to exhaust their limited hospital budget for uncertain cases. I begged them. "Yes, she is too young," I said. "Too young to have us give up. I have exhausted all other means. She has a whole life ahead of her and I cannot help her anymore." I guess that more often than not, I get things done because I am so persistent (though some would use a less flattering description to describe me). I pleaded repeatedly, and Jenny got her SCS trial. For three days she experienced a dramatic reduction in her pain, her leg warmed up, the pain from touching nearly disappeared and she was able to get off the bed and walk without crutches. Seeing these striking results, the neurosurgeons had no other option but to permanently implant the device.

Jenny proved to be one of my most rewarding patients—the kind who makes a doctor's challenging and often difficult life worthwhile. The stimulator continued to work well for years. She finished high school and went on to college. I did not hear from her for at least five years. When her mother called to say I should see her again, I got worried. Thankfully, it turned out I had no reason to be anxious. Jenny had finished college and she was now working full time in a daycare facility. Was she still in chronic pain? "Yes, a bit," she said. "But I did not come for the old pain. I just pulled something in my back lifting a kid and I wanted you to see me." Jenny had turned into an impressively good-looking young woman in her 20s, hair tinted red, slim and trim. I looked at her back. She indeed had some tight muscles in her back, but that was temporary. Her right leg was still sensitive to touch (but just a little). Except for this minor touch pain and a little bit of coldness, she was so much better. She was still using the SCS a few hours most days of the week but she was on no medication. I gave her a few muscle relaxants for her new (muscle) pain and asked her to come back if the new pills did not work. But I guess they did—I never heard from Jenny again. No news is sometimes good news. In my heart I know she is somewhere out there doing well.

Eight

TREATMENTS AND CONTROVERSY

Mention opium to most ordinary people and chances are good that the response will be negative. Most people will likely associate it with vice and sin, addiction and crime. But opium is also the wellspring of a vast branch of pain-relief remedies. And there is strong evidence that people have known of the therapeutic powers of opium for a long, long time.

Opium comes from poppy seeds. The remains of poppy seeds dating back to 4000 B.C. were discovered by Swedish archeologists. In Egypt, the Ebers Papyrus, written in approximately 1550 B.C., includes numerous prescriptions for opium as a medicine for pain. The ancient Greeks and Romans in their writings also mentioned opium and its medical uses. Opium may have been one of the first drugs ever discovered.[1]

From opium itself comes a whole class of drugs that can treat pain effectively—called opioids. Some opioids, such as morphine and codeine, are derived naturally from opium. Others are partially synthesized from opium, as part of their chemical structure occurs naturally, while another part is made in the laboratory. A third type of opioid is totally synthetic, made in the laboratory. Partially synthesized opioids include hydromorphone (known as Dilaudid commercially) and oxycodone (the ingredient of the popular analgesics Percocet and OxyContin). Completely synthetic opioids are meperidine (known as Demerol), fentanyl (found in the popular Duragesic patch that delivers analgesia through the skin) and methadone (used for treatment of heroin addicts as well as for pain).

Morphine was first extracted from opium as a commercially available drug in 1830. From our perspective today, attitudes in the nineteenth century sometimes seem remarkably tolerant toward opium; in Victorian Britain it was used as both sedative and stimulant, and it is mentioned in the Sherlock Holmes stories of Sir Arthur Conan Doyle. At the same time, opium was viewed as problematic; Victorian fiction frequently casts "opium eaters" as criminals. As opium and morphine were proven to be addictive, scientists tried to find a non-addictive alternative, and in 1874 they came up with heroin.

Unfortunately, heroin as well proved to be highly addictive and its manufacture was banned in the United States, though not until 1924. (Interestingly, there were several years in the United States when it was perfectly legal to manufacture heroin but against the law to make beer or wine.) Other opioid drugs appeared in the early to mid-1900s in the West, and were extremely powerful in suppressing pain, but all of them proved to be also highly addictive. By 1900, one American in 200 was either a cocaine or an opium addict, many of them becoming addicted inadvertently through legal medicines. The U.S. Pure Food and Drug Act of 1906 required, for the first time, manufacturers of patent medicines to disclose drug content. Concern about opioids became intense in the 1950s—doctors were extremely uncomfortable with prescribing them because of fear of addiction. Twenty years later, this thinking started changing: where once addiction had been viewed as a psychological phenomenon, it was now seen more as a disorder of chemical imbalance. Once addiction started to be viewed differently, opioids began to be recommended for cancer patients. Particularly when the patient's life expectancy is short, aggressive therapy for palliation of pain is humane and appropriate.

Concerns about addiction still hindered the use of opioids for patients with chronic but non-malignant pain. But in a seminal paper published in the mid-1990s, two well-known scientists working with cancer patients reported that opioids could also help some patients with non-cancer pain.[2] This paper caused a significant shift in medical thinking, promoting much more liberal use of opioids in treating patients, both those with cancer and those whose pain was not caused by cancer.

Today, however, the pendulum has moved from one extreme, that of "opiophobia" to the other extreme, which many call "opiophilia." The advocates and critics have become polarized, and in medical meetings the issue often leaves the realm of scientific discussion to become emotionally charged.[3]

I use opioids extensively in my practice, which concentrates around non-malignant (non-cancer) pain. However, I am very careful and I ask myself many questions before I put a patient on long-term opioids. What is the cause and mechanism of the pain? Is it arthritis? Inflammation? A nerve injury? Depending on the mechanism of pain—how the pain wends its way through the patient's body (and mind), opioids may be ineffective. I also ask: Have other forms of treatment been tried before? What are the benefits of long-term opioid use versus the risks and side effects—possible addiction, dependence, constipation, dizziness and confusion? How is the use of these drugs going to affect the patient's efforts at rehabilitation, since it is easier to subdue the pain with drugs than deal more comprehensively with the complex physical and emotional triggers. And what are the legal implications for me as the prescribing physician and for my patient? What happens, for example, if a patient gets involved in a car accident while driving under the influence of mind-altering drugs that I prescribed?

When it comes to the use of opioids, pain doctors are divided. Physicians like me, who focus on rehabilitation and restoration of function despite limitations, judge the success of opioids by how much a patient can do and how well he or she can operate in his or her environment while using the medication. Others, who focus primarily on pain relief, consider opioids successful if they make the patient feel better by simply easing the pain.

Opioids are highly effective in cases of acute pain after injuries or surgery. There is also no doubt that serious persistent pain in these acute cases can mess up the body's immunity and delay recovery. Opioids are also highly effective in cancer pain. But several questions remain unanswered for non-malignant pain.[4] From the strict scientific point of view, no well-designed studies have been published yet that provide sufficient information about the implications of long-term opioid therapy for non-cancer patients. How effective are these drugs in cases of non-cancer pain? Exactly when is it appropriate to prescribe them and in what doses? What long-term effects do they have? And how do they affect functional recovery in patients with chronic, intractable, non-malignant pain? For all their virtues, opioids are not magic drugs that can address every kind of pain. In some studies, even with liberal application, more than one-third of patients fail to experience pain relief. Different types of pains respond differently to drugs. In particular, studies in people and animals have shown that neuropathic pain is harder to treat and more resistant to opioids.[5]

Another significant issue is the question of addiction. The clinical definition of addiction is the "compulsive use of a substance like alcohol or drugs, illicit or prescribed, resulting in physical, psychological or social injury to the user and continued use despite this harm."[6] Addiction is both a physical and a psychological state. Addicts are psychologically dependent, as they crave the drug for the buzz they get or to avoid the withdrawal effects that occur when the body is deprived of a drug. They are also physically dependent, as abrupt stopping of the addictive drug will produce withdrawal symptoms such as fast heartbeat, cramps, nausea and vomiting, sweating and teary eyes. Patients in chronic pain who use opioids for a long time will develop physical dependence, so if they want to stop the drug they must do it slowly to avoid withdrawal symptoms, but this does not make them addicts. Over time, the body also will probably need increased doses to obtain the same degree of pain relief. In medical terms, this phenomenon, which occurs with opioids, is called "tolerance." In other words, all patients who use opioids chronically will develop physical dependence, and many will develop tolerance. Few, however, will get addicted in the clinical sense. But can we tell in advance which patients are more likely to become addicted?

Research from cancer patients shows that those who use opioids for pain control have only a small risk of becoming addicted. Unfortunately, there are no convincing data so far to show what the risk of addiction is in cases of non-cancer pain. The issue of addiction is poorly addressed in the literature on chronic non-malignant pain, as studies declaring that addiction does not occur in the face of chronic pain are not based on true, clinical measurements of addiction.[7] Yet addiction, in general, is not uncommon. In the United States alone, there are 750,000 to 2 million opioid addicts,[8] and a recent study of a chronic pain clinic showed that drug abuse or addiction occurred in up to one-fifth (18.9 per cent) of patients.[9] The figures contrast sharply with the very low numbers of addicted cancer patients. But even these numbers of addicted non-malignant pain patients that I reported above may not be exact. Doctors, unfortunately, do not have reliable methods to detect patients who are pretending they are in pain or exaggerate their pain complaints in order to obtain narcotics. We really do not know, for example, how common it is for patients to divert medically prescribed drugs to the street for illicit use or profit. Selling opioid drugs can bring big bucks. A 4-milligram tablet of the opioid Dilaudid costs about 75 cents (U.S.) to make but could fetch U.S.$60, while a 10-milligram tablet of OxyContin costing $1.20 sells for U.S.$20 on the street.[10]

Some interesting information regarding the magnitude of abuse of legally prescribed drugs came from the United States Drug Enforcement Administration (DEA), in a talk delivered to the Annual Meeting of the American Pain Society in 2002. According to the DEA records, 2 to 4 per cent of all Americans abuse prescription drugs each year, a number equal to those who abuse cocaine. Both Congress and the DEA are very concerned about one popular opioid, called OxyContin. In Florida more deaths from OxyContin were reported during the first six months in 2001 than from cocaine or heroin. Similarly, in a six-month period, the Boston area experienced 36 violent robberies of pharmacies involving theft of OxyContin, while in North Carolina the DEA officers discovered a ring of criminals who used computer-forged prescriptions to divert large amounts of OxyContin to drug abusers. However, the popular myth that the DEA will prosecute general physicians who prescribe opioids does not seem to hold true, according to the DEA records. During 2001, more than 900,000 doctors in the U.S. were registered as prescribers of controlled substances (including opioids). However, only 861 investigations were undertaken, resulting in 697 actions against violators. Ninety per cent or more of these investigations were initiated through complaints of pharmacists, family members, law enforcement officers or state authorities, for possible illegal activity and diversion of legally prescribed drugs.

Despite all the risks and benefits of prescribing opioids, problematic use or outright addiction seems to happen only in a few situations and in certain patient groups. For example, patients recovering from serious burns who use large doses of opioids do not seem to develop addiction problems.[11] Addiction in the face of chronic pain depends very much on both internal—psychological and personality-related—factors and external ones, such as family, friends and work environment. A great deal was learned about the importance of psychosocial factors in addiction from Vietnam veterans returning home after the war. A whopping 25 per cent of those veterans became addicted to narcotics while in Vietnam, but only 1 per cent continued to use narcotics and considered themselves addicted when they returned to the United States. This shows that when removed from the conditions of severe stress, depression, isolation and an environment in which almost everyone else is on drugs, few people will stick with the habit.[12]

Addiction in the face of chronic pain should be understood in this complex biological/psychological/social context. Regardless of the physical origin of pain, those who suffer from depression, anxiety and extreme stress, and those who are within a certain milieu that supports the use of drugs, are much more likely to use opioids in a problematic way or become addicted.

This context raises several problems for a physician like me when considering prescribing opioids. I have to determine who will benefit from those drugs and who is likely to get into trouble. I must tell the difference between the addict and the one who legitimately will use opioids to subdue the pain. I must be careful when I look at "drug-seeking behaviour" to discriminate the one who seeks the buzz from the person who seeks true pain relief. Indeed, some pain patients seem to possess the same persistent behaviours characteristic of addicts—demanding medications, consuming their prescriptions more quickly than they should, quarrelling with the health care providers and so on. Often, though, these poor souls have been given less medication than they need for their pain. In such cases, once they reach a level of adequate relief, the behaviour ceases.

Several of my patients have pain with causes that are beyond medical or surgical repair. It is these patients who may truly need opioids. Terry, 45, developed severe scoliosis ("crooked spine") at the age of 16. She underwent extensive surgery to stop the progression of the abnormal curvature. This surgery was no small thing. The doctors put a couple of long metal rods with hooks along the length of several vertebrae to fuse the spine and they managed to stop the worsening of the scoliosis. However, as the years passed by, the discs above and below the fusion wore out. Terry found herself in serious pain that hindered her everyday activities.

Around 1999, she had to go on a disability pension, as she was unable to work. Years earlier, Terry had lived with an abusive and alcoholic husband, who drew her deep into alcohol addiction herself. But later, before she stopped working, she had found the courage to walk out of this damaging relationship. She met a wonderful man who fell in love with her and helped her conquer her addiction.

By the time they landed at the doorstep of my clinic, Terry and her new man, Jules, were planning to get married in a few months. They did not ask for much, just for Terry to be able to live with some quality of life and to accompany Jules on his motorcycle rides (he was a diehard Harley-Davidson aficionado). Jules said to me with a sad smile, "My bike is collecting dust in the garage because I don't have what it takes to ride without Terry." How could I not be charmed! But Terry's back was beyond repair. Aspirin-like drugs, physiotherapy, a lumbar support and all kinds of local treatments and even injections had failed. Surgery, too, was out of the question, as Terry's back had been extensively fused—there was not much spine left to operate on. My only option was opioids. I wanted to start Terry with small doses of quick-acting morphine a few times a day, trying to bring the medication to a level where she would have low levels of pain and few or no side effects. Once I figured out how much she needed to function well with the least possible side effects, I would switch her to slow-release morphine, so she would have to take her pill twice or three times a day instead of many times per day.

In considering these opioids for Terry, I had many alternatives—quick- and slow-release morphine; other opioids in pill, liquid or suppository form; and even a skin patch that she would have to change only once every three days. But when I talked to her about my plans, Terry was petrified: "I had such a hard time kicking away the booze a few years ago. I do not want to get hooked now on this." I took my time to explain the risks and the benefits of opioids. I told her that these types of drugs will probably make her body dependent on them and she will get withdrawal symptoms if the drug gets abruptly cut off (the state of "physical dependence" I described earlier). While physical dependence develops in all opioid drug users, and tolerance in many, addiction does not set in unless the single most important determinant of addiction, the psychological component, comes into play. In my estimation Terry was fairly safe—she had a strong will, a good partner, a happy life and realistic expectations. The way she felt about herself and life and her immediate supportive environment seemed good safeguards against developing psychological dependence and addiction. I was vigilant with her, given her previous history of abuse, but I did not deprive her of what she really needed. I finally convinced her. Today, Terry's quality of life has improved substantially with fairly modest doses of slow-release opioids.

I believe I have as many difficulties curtailing inordinate and inappropriate use of opioids as I have in convincing patients with little or no addiction potential that they are safe and should use these valuable drugs. We pain doctors often encounter two kinds of difficult patients who use large doses of opioids: those who continue to suffer from severe pain despite the fact they receive extraordinary doses of morphine or the like (in the order of thousands of milligrams per day), prescribed by well-meaning but extremely liberal and at times ignorant or naive physicians, and those patients who seek drugs. The first group of patients are non-responders to conventional opioids. When it comes to the second group, I admit that no matter how experienced I am, I have been deceived by certain patients who master the art of pretense.

I will not forget Dwight, an executive at a manufacturing company in Northern Ontario whom I saw in the early 1990s for severe pain in his left arm. Before he came to me, he had undergone a couple of surgeries to the ulnar nerve, responsible for the sensation and the motor movements of parts of the forearm and the hand. Dwight was in his late 30s, married with two kids. Reluctantly, I put him on modest doses of a narcotic I rarely prescribe (Leritine), after everything else we tried did not seem to work. I did not mind him using a few pills a day as he was working full time and appeared to have a stable life. He was actually okay for several years, but things changed when the factory was sold to a U.S. company. Dwight was given two years to turn the books around and make the money-losing operation profitable, or it would be shut down. The family doctor referred him back to me—he had not been under my care for more than three years—because his pain was getting worse. When my team examined Dwight, our view was that he was depressed and stressed out from his 15-hours-a-day, 7-days-a-week work schedule. It was obvious to us what Dwight needed to do to relieve his pain: change his lifestyle, manage his stress and look beyond opioids to deal with his anxiety and depression. Dwight, however, did not seem to value our suggestions, and odd things started happening. Dwight once came to ask for a copy of my files, as he said he was searching for a new physician since his family practitioner was moving out of town. A month later I got an urgent call from his wife that Dwight had lost his suitcase on a recent trip, along with his pain medications. She said the local family physician was sick and he had no replacement. Did I mind just giving him a week's prescription "to tide him over?" Losing prescriptions or medications is a common trick of drug addicts, so I had to be careful. We phoned the local doctor's office and the call was picked up by an answering machine, which did not indicate that the departing physician was being replaced. So I gave Dwight a week's prescription.

A month later I got a call from an insurance doctor who was looking over Dwight's prescriptions submitted for repayment by his company drug plan. Did I know, the doctor asked, that Dwight was receiving the same pills from not one, but three, doctors at the same time? He faxed me the prescriptions. To my dismay, Dwight had two general practitioners and me simultaneously prescribing a total of 56 tablets of Leritine per day—instead of the six per day that I was giving him myself. "By the way," the insurance doctor added, "did you also know that one of these family practitioners (one I was not even aware of previously) has also been prescribing 300 tablets of the same drug every month to Dwight's wife?"

I was outraged, as I felt deceived and used. Dwight and his wife were due for a visit the next week. They came in, well dressed as usual, emotions under control, polite and sophisticated. With a calm face and a steady voice I asked Dwight what the name of the other practitioner (the one he had never mentioned to me) meant to him. An awkward silence followed. "You see, I told you we have a problem," his wife said. She knew the game was over. Dwight asked me if I knew a drug treatment centre (whose information I provided) and if I was willing to take him back to my care after he had undergone treatment (which I said I would). The couple left with profuse apologies. I notified the other practitioners of what I knew.

Dwight never returned to my care. I found out later that he never returned to the care of the other two doctors either. Who else is he scamming now for narcotics? Dwight's triple doctoring was caught by a silly mistake of his— submitting prescriptions for reimbursement for the same drug ordered by three different physicians. Ontario and many other provinces in Canada do not have safeguards to catch double and triple doctoring. By comparison, Manitoba has a triplicate prescription system. One prescription copy stays with the doctor, the second one with the pharmacy and the third one is sent to a central registry. Some physicians fear that this type of rigourous system would lead to their prosecution if double or triple doctoring is discovered. But I have no doubt that such a system would spare me and many other physicians the grief of having patients like Dwight.

Multiple emergency visits, insistence that only one specific kind of drug works (most times they ask for it by name), appearances at the doctor's office for lost or stolen prescriptions and double or triple doctoring are not unusual for abusers. Years ago a patient signed himself out of my in-patient unit when we insisted that he submit to urine and blood sample analysis. The team's consensus was that he had drug-seeking behaviour. Our conclusion was based on a number of signs—the multiple complaints he had for which we could find no medical explanation, his frequent emergency visits for injections of Demerol, his aggressive and argumentative behaviour and his refusal to co-operate during the tests. It ended up that he did to me and others what is every practising physician's nightmare. He sent a huge letter of complaint (37 handwritten pages) to my professional governing body, the College of Physicians and Surgeons of Ontario, contending that three physicians and I did not appropriately address his pain. An investigation was initiated, which meant I had to copy all my files, supply my side of the story and spend a significant amount of time away from my patients just to address the questions of the investigator of the College. At least I did not have to hire a lawyer. Nine months later the investigation concluded that the complainant was triple-doctoring and forging prescriptions. All four of us were exonerated, but after considerable aggravation and waste of time.

Ron, who is 45, was sent to me recently by his family practitioner. Unfortunately, the only information I was given about his history was scribbled in a handwritten note by the referring physician. Ron confused me a great deal as he gave me a long, convoluted history of severe injuries and medical ailments, which led to several surgical interventions. As I was talking to him, the dates, types of surgeries and reasons for his surgeries were different from those the physician had recorded in his note. Some years ago (it could be 1992 or 1996 Ron said, but he could not exactly remember), he fell off the wing of a plane when he was working at the airport (he was unclear if it was in Toronto or Detroit) and injured himself. The note said he suffered a complex fracture of the left shoulder, but Ron told me he had had a neck surgery. I finally figured out that the neck surgery was dated 1999. Before or after that, according to Ron, he also had three back surgeries, which included a fusion and the insertion of metal rods in his back. Maybe in 1998 (he was not sure about this either) Ron underwent surgery on his left hip, because it had been "shattered" for reasons I could not figure out and which he could not explain.

In March 2001, Ron said he had some benign (non-cancerous) growth removed from his rib cage. The physician's note stated, however, that this was an infection of the ribs. As if all his surgeries were not enough, over the last few years Ron said he was developing abscesses (cavities with pus) all over his body. Again the physician's note did not mention any such thing. Ron was asked to shade in where he was feeling pain on a drawing of his body. He shaded in almost every part of his back, neck, hips, legs and head.

Ron was a "customer" of a private "block" clinic. This particular clinic was extremely well known for its liberal (and, I believe, indiscriminate) use of "nerve blocks"—injections of freezing sometimes mixed with cortisone into the path of small skin nerves or into the muscles. This clinic and similar ones perform thousands of nerve blocks every year. Their patients visit regularly, in many cases every week, for many weeks in a row, and they are often given several injections each time. Even worse, often the patients are first submitted to general anaesthesia (otherwise they would not be able to tolerate 10 to 12 injections at a time) and when they wake up, they are given some handfuls of opioids to combat the pain from the injections, until relief comes (which sometimes never occurs). Although nerve blocks have their place in certain chronic pain cases, the regular long-term use of such injections without persistent benefit is not a practice supported by what we know in the scientific literature.[13] Sophisticated clinics often associated with universities (mine is an example) are conservative and careful in the use of nerve blocks, which they reserve for carefully selected patients, while some private clinics and certain physicians seem to use them extremely liberally. Often at the root of such an abused technique is money. The more injections a patient is given, the more money the doctor and the facility bill the system (which for Canada as a whole is fee-for-service).

Ron was a regular customer in such a private clinic, which also fed him inordinate amounts of narcotics in the form of injections many times a day. He was actually given enough supply to inject himself at home with an opioid called Dilaudid (hydromorphone) every four hours, the equivalent of 1800 milligrams of oral morphine a day. At times he was using more than twice this amount, roughly 4 grams of morphine daily. Despite these doses, Ron rated his pain as 9 out of 10 on my pain scale, and he complained that the medication was not really making it any better. He added that he was very upset because this block clinic "turned him into a junkie," claiming that he himself never wanted these medications. He said he had "never used drugs or pot himself." He was not convincing.

Ron boasted that he owned his own company, manufacturing "high-performance cars." He said he was the president and had several employees. He proudly told me that he owned 13 Porsches. I must admit that Ron's scruffy appearance and unshaven face was far from the picture of an executive in my mind. His body looked somehow twisted as he was walking, stooped and stiff. Deep irregular scars marked his arms, looking like recently cultivated farmland, scars that he said were due to several infections. Long scars as well marked his spine and his chest wall, while the skin along his abdomen looked broken down, apparently the result of significant weight loss. He said that he had lost 45 kilograms (100 pounds) in the last five years. Despite all this Ron insisted he was not depressed, and as far as sex was concerned he stated, "he was tending to his business properly with the wife." For all this boasting, on examination it was his neck, back and hips that were stiff. Ron sighed and grimaced and held his back and complained of pain during the visit, while he winced at the mere touch of my fingertip throughout his whole body.

I thought: What a story! I told Ron that I was sorry, but I was not prepared to do anything until I could receive information for my files. I wanted to see hospital records and surgical notes, X-rays and other tests that he said he had. Ron "was surprised," as he said he knew all his files had been mailed to my office weeks before. I wrote to his family physician asking about further files (if he actually had any). In my consult note I expressed grave concern for the inordinate amount of injectable narcotics, particularly when his pain was not responding at all. I left it there. I seriously doubted that Ron intended to visit me again. I was right. He never showed up again and to this date no more of his files have reached my desk.

Over the past three years my practice has changed drastically. No week goes by now without me seeing patients who are obviously taking large and unjustified doses of narcotics. They come in all forms and shapes; sophisticated executives like Dwight; hard-core addicts with scarred arms and scruffy faces like Ron; innocent-looking grandmas; booze-smelling ex-cons; young, beautiful, educated women; all in pain, real, imaginary or pretend. The common source of referral is their family physicians. Some of these doctors feel stuck with patients who demand narcotics, which they are uncomfortable prescribing. Other physicians had taken it upon themselves to prescribe opioids liberally until they became worried by new professional rules; my governing body, the College of Physicians and Surgeons of Ontario, brought in new regulations recently. [14] The College is the regulatory body responsible for the medical license of the nearly 20,000 doctors in my province, equivalent to Medical Boards in the United States. In mid-1996, the College asked me and six other pain physicians who are known for their expertise and research skills to create a set of guidelines for doctors regarding good chronic pain practices. It took our team four years of complex work, and finally, in November 2000, the College accepted our work and approved North America's first "evidence-based recommendations for the medical management of chronic non-malignant pain." Our work was dispassionate—we avoided saying what we personally liked or disliked in pain management. Rather, we produced a consolidated review of the best literature in chronic pain and a summary of what has been found to work or not work, based on extensive research. Among other topics, the guidelines addressed, at great length, the issue of chronic opioid use in non-malignant pain. After the publication of these guidelines the doctors in the province had some kind of a roadmap to guide them on how to manage patients on opioids. I served as co-chair of the group that produced these guidelines, and I think that's one reason why I ended up seeing so many patients who have been using opioids in a problematic way. However, when I talk to other colleagues in reputable pain clinics, they say they face similar problems to mine.

On the other hand, approximately 40 per cent or more of my patients truly *need* opioids. Often I have as much trouble convincing worthy patients to take these valuable drugs as I have taking those who abuse them off the medication. Similarly, while some physicians give out opioids indiscriminately and in large doses, many more doctors, afraid of their patients becoming addicted or of "persecution" by the College, deny the benefit of opioids to their patients even in small doses. So what kind of patients am I prepared to place on narcotics and why?

Marilyn, now 32, suffers from a rare genetic disease called neurofibromatosis, which is characterized by café-au-lait-coloured spots on the skin and minuscule skin lumps, along with many tumours that grow on nerves and nerve roots. Marilyn was sent to us some four years ago by her neurosurgeons for severe and persistent mid-back pain, which radiated out to her neck and right arm. They had planned surgery for her, unless we could come up with an easier treatment. Years before, she had had a couple of tumours removed from her cervical spine to avoid compression of her spinal cord. Marilyn also had severe deformity of her spine (kyphoscoliosis), which caused her head to deviate to the right. She complained that her pain was shooting and aching in her upper back and became worse with activities. Actually, she could point exactly to where she hurt, she said.

When she undressed, Marilyn proved to be a textbook case of neurofibromatosis. She allowed me to take several pictures of her body (covering her face, of course, for reasons of privacy and confidentiality). The most remarkable thing about Marilyn, however, was not the spots and the numerous skin tags all over her flesh . . . but a bizarre and indescribable mass of something hard around her left shoulder, which was higher than the right one. For the life of me, I could not tell if this was fibrous tissue or bone. X-rays and a CAT scan gave me the answer. Marilyn's severely twisted spine had caused her left shoulder blade to be rotated and pushed forward. This was the hard stuff I was feeling under my fingers. On top of it, her upper shoulder muscles had shrunk and shortened into tight fibrous bands sitting over the hump.

I thought Marilyn's pain was coming from this bony deformity and the imbalance of muscles, and had nothing to do with her neurological condition, so surgery was not warranted. For two years she did well with a couple of tablets of Percocet, a short-acting narcotic that she used to take only when she needed it. More recently, as her kyphoscoliosis has progressed, there are days when she needs four Percocets (which I gladly prescribe). She is able to respond to small doses of narcotics, as her pain is nociceptive in origin (usually these pains respond very well to opioids). Marilyn's quality of life is substantially improved, as she is able to attend part-time classes and have a reasonable social life. Most importantly, the surgery that was originally planned for her never took place.

Fred was 39 when he was referred to me. His ordeal began when, at the age of 24, he developed arthritis and swelling in his left big toe. This was diagnosed as psoriatic arthritis (a form of severe, destructive arthritis) and it soon spread to other joints. By the time he was 36, his hip joints were so damaged that they were both replaced by artificial ones. Two years later, both his knees needed replacement surgery as well. During Fred's prolonged and difficult knee surgeries, pressure over his legs damaged the nerves at the back of each of his calves. By the time he came to the clinic he was severely depressed to the point that he wanted to kill himself. His pain was unbearable. Ankles, hands, elbows, neck and back were all constantly hurting, with pain he described as deep, aching and gnawing. The nerve injury pain was different, with a shooting and stabbing sensation that went into his calves and feet. Fred was on strong medication for the inflammation caused by his arthritis but no analgesic medication for his pains except over-the-counter Tylenol. His ankles were severely twisted and deformed and his feet were splayed and flat. Fred's wrists and elbows were in no better shape. I offered him some small doses of a quick-acting form of morphine called Statex.

I explained to Fred that he suffered from two types of pain—nociceptive pain caused by the severe arthritis and neuropathic pain because of the nerve damage. I told him that to control his pains, he needed to take opioid analgesics around the clock. But Fred was hesitant. "I am afraid I will get addicted," he said. "Besides, I would like to keep morphine only as my last resort." Here we go again, I thought. I took time to explain to him the differences between addiction, physical dependence and tolerance, and I managed to persuade Fred to follow my advice. He left with a prescription of 5 milligrams of Statex every four hours (a "baby" dose). Six weeks later Fred came back for follow-up. His overall pain had subsided dramatically. He was capable of doing more about his personal care and looking after his life. Fred managed to attend his cousin's wedding—something he would not have been able to do before—and he did quite well throughout the evening. His mood reflected this dramatic improvement. Altogether his pain ratings had dropped from 7 out of 10 down to 2, on a mere 25 milligrams of Statex a day, a dose 100 to 200 times smaller than the one used by Ron, whose pain ratings continued to be 9.

This is not to say that all people respond the same way to a given amount of morphine. Research has shown without doubt that large differences exist between individuals in the way the body handles narcotics. But I have learned one thing during my two decades of practice: patients with solid physical pathology and a stable personality, good coping skills and a supportive environment may need much less medication than patients whose behavioural and psychological problems complicate the picture. I switched Fred to equivalent doses of slow-release morphine preparations. So far, he has been doing well. However, my intervention is not going to change the nature of his arthritis or the serious destruction of his joints. Sooner or later, Fred will require more surgery, and gradually his needs for morphine will increase, but he will probably still remain on relatively small doses of opioids.

There are physicians who feel that "all pains will go away if only the patient can get enough opioids." It is not unusual to see daily prescriptions of large doses of morphine, in the thousands of milligrams. I consider myself to be a "middle of the road" physician in this regard. I feel that most patients (depending on the underlying pain mechanisms) can obtain substantial relief with morphine in doses of less than 300 milligrams per day. At times, of course, I will exceed this dose by far, but for few, specific patients and only for specific pain mechanisms—for example, for patients with a broken spine after an accident who end up paralyzed, or for patients with damage to the nerves that innervate their limbs or the pelvic and abdominal viscera.

The guidelines my group developed for the College of Physicians and Surgeons of Ontario[15] advise that when a patient requires "morphine megadoses," the prescribing physician should take a moderate, "common sense" approach, in particular attaching careful consideration to three potential reasons as to why so much drug may be required:

1. The patient may not be able to absorb or metabolize the drug. For example, 7 to 10 per cent of all Caucasians have a defective gene that produces a non-functional enzyme called P450IID6. This enzyme is responsible for the metabolism of at least 40 widely used drugs, including the powerful analgesic codeine. Since the individuals who carry this gene are unable to convert codeine into morphine, they may consume large quantities of the drug, yet still feel serious pain.[16]

2. The patient may suffer from a type of pain that does not respond to opioids. For example, neuropathic pain is notoriously resistant to narcotics. This is not to say it does not respond at all, but the patient needs larger doses to experience good relief. As a matter of fact, most patients of mine with serious neuropathic pain cannot do without morphine or other opioids. Simply, they need larger doses than, for example, a patient with serious hip arthritis. On the other hand, patients with serious psychological problems not only run a higher risk of addiction, but they may take megadoses of morphine without much effect.

3. Certain patients who take huge amounts of narcotics may "divert" them or sell them for profit, as the DEA and other statistics show.

If used wisely, opioids can make a huge difference in a chronic-pain patient's life. They may be exactly what helps patients get out of bed, go shopping, get around to doing personal things, fulfill their role as a wife or husband and go to work. I was called some years ago to see a 70-year-old woman with severe spinal stenosis, a severe narrowing of the bony spine caused by degenerated discs and resulting in compression of the long nerves that go down the legs. So Mama Michaela, as everyone called her, could not take care of her little house nor could she go shopping. She lived alone. The doctors did not want to operate on her because of her age and the severity of her disease.

Her daughter was very concerned. She was living in another city, travelling constantly for work, and her only alternative was to place her mother in a seniors' home.

Mama Michaela despised the idea. She loved her little bungalow and her miniature garden. "I have no stairs, Doctor," she said. "My neighbour could take me shopping once a week, if I could only walk a few blocks. Can you do something to help me with this back and leg pain?" Physiotherapy had not helped Mama and Aspirin-like drugs were quite hard on her stomach. I put her on small doses of quick-release morphine. I advised her to take the pills "around the clock" every four hours and to keep a pain diary. She was quite lucid, sharp as a knife. I did not want to dull her brains, or make her dizzy, fall and break her hip (which could be fatal at her age). I advised her to increase the fibre in her diet to combat constipation, and I sent her off with a return appointment in three weeks.

When she returned, Mama Michaela came alone, without her daughter. She had a big smile. "What a difference, Doctor. I can do my shopping now, and I can even walk with my neighbour's daughter to the park. I have only one problem that bothers me. I can't make it here every month or two to get my new prescription, and my doctor is afraid that he will lose his licence if he prescribes what you are giving me."

Unfortunately, Mama Michaela was not the only patient to have this experience. Some family practitioners with limited knowledge of how to manage chronic pain would adamantly refuse to follow my advice and renew the prescription of opioids for patients who my clinic feels could benefit from this class of drugs. That is terribly hard on those patients who may have to travel a long distance to see us, and to a lesser extent for us, in that we have to play the role of primary-care physician for hundreds of patients, which diverts us from the care people count on us to provide. In this situation, I try to educate the physicians by sending them a summary of the College's guidelines, as well as assuring them that I and the other members of my clinic will always be around to help out. In the worst situations, I advise the patient to change family doctors. In Michaela's case, her physician turned out to be receptive to my suggestions. I switched her to slow-release morphine preparations and I saw her a few more times to make sure everything was working well. Her doctor felt comfortable with the literature I sent to him and my telephone explanations, and since our exchange he has continued to prescribe what Michaela needs.

Over the last few years, as physicians have become more at ease with the use of opioids for chronic non-malignant pain, we have also discovered opioids other than morphine that have special properties and can help certain kinds of patients. Methadone, for example, is a completely synthetic opioid, well known in the treatment of addicts. It is also a powerful analgesic for cancer pain. It is long-acting, as it stays in the body for days rather than hours. It also works particularly well for a certain kind of opioid receptor, the *delta* receptors. When a patient's *mu* receptors (the ones responding to morphine) become resistant to the morphine, methadone can provide extra pain relief. Methadone also acts against specific receptors that are active in patients with neuropathic pain. This drug in certain patients may produce lesser side effects (such as nausea and vomiting) than other opioids. It is only in the last few years that methadone has been used for non-malignant pain. In Ontario and other provinces in Canada, a physician needs a special licence to prescribe methadone.

Methadone still has a long way to go in pain management. Physicians in Ontario with a licence to prescribe this drug for drug addicts do not necessarily know much about chronic pain. Doctors have to be educated if they are to manage chronic pain effectively with methadone. At the same time, many patients have to be educated as well, as they often refuse the drug, protesting that they are not drug addicts. They need to understand that this is not the only reason we prescribe methadone.

For all the discussion of the pros and the cons of long-term opioid use in chronic pain, the jury is still out. In terms of psychological issues, studies show that opioids can worsen depression and produce anxiety and irritability.[17] Patients' families often complain that patients on chronic opioid therapy are jittery and get angry easily. Pain patients, whether the pain is cancer-related or not, can be slower in their reaction times and somewhat confused, specifically when they are in the process of changing doses or when they take extra opioids (what we call a "rescue" dose) for a flare-up of their pain.[18]

Another important issue relates to the cost, or possibly the cost savings, of opioid use for our health care services. Do patients with chronic non-malignant pain on long-term opioid therapy save the system money by using health care services less frequently (whether these services are publicly funded, as in Canada and Europe, or privately funded, as in the United States)? Studies suggest the contrary. Long-term opioid patients are more likely to be hospitalized more frequently, undergo more surgeries, spend more money on prescriptions, take other medications to which they also become dependent (like medicines for anxiety or insomnia) and end up requiring additional drugs to combat the side effects of opioids. This may relate to the severity of the underlying condition that led to the administration of opioids. On the other hand, use of opioids (at times in large doses) instead of other pharmacological or nonmedicinal treatments that could be useful in pain control can be associated with side effects that prompt patients to use the health care system more.[19]

Chronic opioid use also raises serious issues of liability and insurability in our litigious society. The issue of driving ability in particular has received quite a bit of attention in the medical literature.[20] I have many patients on chronic opioid therapy, and I worry when they are on increasing doses of opioids or when they take extra (rescue) doses and they then have to drive, operate heavy machinery or do jobs where a high level of attention or serious decision-making is needed. How comfortable can I feel when a patient on high-dose opioids may be someone driving my kids to school or operating a crane overhead or even preparing my tax return? I am not the only one who worries about these issues. Many of my patients worry too. Most of them won't drive, particularly if they are on high doses of opioids. Some who maintain full-time work will refuse to take their medications during their working day and will take them only when they return home. Even given these concerns, I don't worry so much if they are stable on low to modest doses. To the contrary, I have good reason to believe that serious and untreated pain clouds my patients' brains much more than modest doses of opioids will. Each one of the patients on opioids must be seen as a unique case, and these issues should be discussed with both the patient and his or her family. To the best of my knowledge, no specific guidelines or even tests exist that would let my patients be tested reliably, for example, by the Ministry of Transportation in my province. Nevertheless, I suspect that eventually this will change, as we must find better ways of determining who should be able to take opioids beneficially and drive or perform other activities that require attention, concentration and co-ordination.

Controversy and debate about the use of opioids in chronic pain will continue. Today, more than ever, the heat is on. In this country and the United States, polarized and sensational media often look at opioids without presenting scientific data and expert and scientific testimonies. While the medical community remains divided and regulatory bodies in many cases offer confusing, conflicting advice, opioids will continue to draw attention in the media and in public debates. As the scientific community takes a more active role in trying to establish appropriate do's and don'ts, I anticipate that eventually the pendulum will settle in the middle, and opioids will be given carefully to those who truly need the drugs and will benefit, while physicians will become even more at ease with prescribing these medications for suitable patients.

To Smoke or Not to Smoke: Medical Marijuana

About a year ago, I received an urgent request from a nursing home administrator to see one of the home's patients. For the first time I came face to face with a new breed of pain patients: those who request the doctor's blessing to smoke pot for medical reasons.

Carl was 36 and had made this particular nursing home his permanent residence for the previous five years, ever since he suffered a severe stroke after long use of free-base cocaine. The right side of his body was paralyzed and his slurred speech was difficult to understand. Carl had some kind of pain in his left hip, whose cause nobody could figure out. It seemed that nothing worked for this pain . . . except marijuana. The unusual problem the administrator had was that Carl's father was bringing pot into the nursing home and despite repeated warnings by the management, Carl was caught several times smoking in his room. The questions the nursing home administrator asked me were: Could I find the origin of Carl's pain? Could I suggest some alternatives for pain management? Smoking of all sorts was strictly prohibited in the home and smoking marijuana has been in general illegal in Canada.

Carl came to my clinic in an ambulance, on a stretcher and accompanied by his attentive father. He needed help to turn around in bed. He was wearing an adult diaper because he had little bladder control. But he was able to answer some of our questions. He said he had "lots of pain" and pointed vaguely across his left hip. Every attempt to move the hip generated strong pain reactions. However, when Carl's attention was distracted by one of my assistants who was examining his shoulders, I was able to move his hip freely and even press hard on it without the slightest sign of discomfort. Such examination "under distraction" tells me a lot. Real physical pain due to inflammation, arthritis or other physical causes may be less intense when attention is switched to something else, but does not disappear. Moving the hip vigorously should have jolted Carl's attention and brought him back to reality . . . and pain. But X-rays of the hip and a bone scan showed no abnormalities. I was convinced that Carl's pain had no physical origin, and in my books he had no medical justification to use pot. As a matter of fact, he had no medical reason to need opioids or any other kind of strong painkillers.

Unfortunately, Carl was typical of the patients who are referred to my clinic with the question of medical use of marijuana to be answered. Most of these patients had been habitual users of pot and other drugs before the onset of their medical affliction. In Carl's case, the father proved as resistant as the son when one of my colleagues who specializes in pain and chemical dependence discussed alternatives. Carl and his father turned down the offer of pills containing the active ingredient of marijuana, Delta-9-THC (tetrahydrocannabinol). Carl blatantly admitted that he needed his buzz, and the pills do not provide this, as they have a slow and unpredictable absorption through the stomach. By inhaling the smoke, the drug bypasses the stomach and THC hits the brain directly, as the drug enters the bloodstream fast.

The *cannabis sativa L* or hemp plant was one of the first plants to be used by humans to create fibres, food and medicines and in social and religious rituals. It grows in almost every part in the world. In most fibre-producing areas the plant is used only for the manufacture of clothes and ropes, as climate and ground factors affect the content of the pharmacologically active ingredients that are responsible for the mood-altering effects of marijuana. Cannabis was used by the Yellow Emperor, or Huang-Ti, (around 2600 B.C.) for its medicinal and mood-altering effects and as an anaesthetic in wine for major operations around the third century A.D.[21] It was also used by the Assyrians, the Sumerians and many other ancient civilizations for pain, inflammation, epilepsy and various other diseases. Historically, in India, the plant was used both medically and non-medically. On a few social occasions, the weaker preparation of the plant called *bhang* (comparable to marijuana) was taken by mouth, while slightly stronger preparations (*ganja*) were smoked. Hashish, the strongest preparation of all, was used in the Middle East and Asia, but like marijuana itself, its use has long been controversial. Known as *charas* in India, it was not socially approved there for any purposes, and those who used it were regarded as "bad people" or outcasts.[22]

When it comes specifically to the treatment of pain, cannabinoids were used by ancient populations thousands of years ago, as well as by Asian populations in the Middle Ages and for different pains in the West during the 1800s, with commercial preparations supplied by the pharmaceutical companies Lilly and Squibb. However, cannabinoids were discontinued as medical agents in the 1930s.[23] It was only in 1964 that the sole psychoactive ingredient of cannabis, Delta-9-THC (tetrahydrocannabinol), was isolated in pure form. The discovery of morphine receptors in the brain and the spinal cord in the 1970s led to the discovery of endorphins, the body's own painkillers. Similarly, the discovery of cannabinoid receptors in the brain (primarily CB1) raised the question of whether the brain produces marijuana-like substances as well. Indeed, two such internally produced compounds, called *endocannabinoids*, were discovered. After that discovery, synthetic cannabinoids were created, some of which have other than psychoactive functions. For the following 20 years, thousands of papers appeared on the chemical, pharmacological, metabolic and clinical aspects of cannabinoids in animals and humans. Today, synthetic cannabinoids are used to increase the appetite of patients with AIDS and for prevention of vomiting and nausea in cancer patients who are undergoing chemotherapy. After some successful experiments in animals, studies of people with brain injury are now under way in Europe, as it seems that certain cannabinoids help protect the nervous tissue from damage. Another cannabinoid seems to act against inflammation and anxiety and has been tried on patients with epilepsy. Numerous animal experiments show as well that cannabinoids can block many different kinds of pains, so there is little doubt today that cannabinoids are inhibiting pain transmission.

The question we face now is not whether cannabinoids can be marketed as drugs for people. They already are: drugs that are commercially available in the form of pills include dronabinol (commercially known as Marinol in Canada and elsewhere) and nabilone (known as Cesamet). The current hot debate in medical and political circles relates to the question of whether *smoking* marijuana for medical reasons should be permitted, as smoking in general carries major risks for inflammation of our lungs and lung cancer. The U.S. National Academy of Sciences Institute of Medicine, recognizing that smoking in general is associated with grave health risks, recommended in 1999 that therapeutic uses of smoked marijuana be highly regulated and reserved for "dire circumstances."[24] The issue would seem to end there on medical grounds, but unfortunately, there is a serious drawback with the use of pills because they are absorbed slowly and unpredictably. The pills may indeed produce pain relief, but they can also have bad effects on mood, so they are not that useful. Certain laboratories are now trying to develop other forms of delivering the active ingredients of marijuana to the blood instead of pills, or to create other compounds that do not affect the mood while they block pain. Furthermore, scientists are actively working to find new drugs that may increase the synthesis of the body's own cannabinoids or impair their breakdown. Adding these other drugs may increase pain relief, especially in cases where opioids do not work well or produce unacceptable side effects.[25]

It is worth discussing the views of respectable international medical bodies before we can understand the dilemma we doctors face in places like Canada as far as the decriminalization of marijuana for medical use is concerned. Major reviews of the possible therapeutic actions of cannabinoids have been conducted in Great Britain, Australia and the United States. All of these major reports consider smoking unacceptable except in special circumstances, such as when patients are terminally ill with short life expectancy, or in other cases for a limited time only. All suggest research into alternative methods of administration of the active ingredient for rapid action without the risks associated with smoke inhalation. They all accept, as well, that cannabinoids have special actions against nausea, vomiting, lack of appetite, pain and spasticity and recommend clinical trials. Most medical communities feel that proper studies are needed before the general use of cannabis or cannabinoids could be recommended.[26]

However, in Canada the issue of medical access to marijuana reached a legal milestone on July 30, 2001, when, following a highly publicized Supreme Court of Canada case, the federal government hastily established a set of Marijuana Medical Access Regulations. These regulations spelled out three categories of people who can apply to possess marijuana for medical reasons:

1. People who suffer from a terminal illness and are doomed to die within 12 months.
2. Those who suffer from specific symptoms, such as pain, spasms, nausea and so on, which are related to particular diseases such as multiple sclerosis, spinal cord diseases, AIDS or severe arthritis, provided that all other available treatments have been tried and found not to be appropriate.
3. Those suffering from conditions other than those in the first two categories, provided again that all other treatments have failed.

Patients in the first and second groups require a declaration from one medical specialist. Patients in the third group require declarations from two doctors. A lengthy form, many pages long, can be obtained from the Health Canada website as well as a guide with regulations and explanations for the application process, for patients who want to either grow their own pot or have someone grow it for them.

In my view, our politicians in Canada jumped the gun and placed the cart before the horse. Bending to political and lobbying powers, they passed the issue from their shoulders to the shoulders of the medical profession. For the first time, doctors are asked to prescribe a drug for which we are unable to look for information, indications, contraindications, dosages and so on. For pot, we must acknowledge when we sign this very long form the patients bring us that we know that the drug has not been tested for safety and effectiveness. We must also declare that "the benefits . . . outweigh any risks associated with its use." But how can I tell patients about risks and benefits when I do not know them and when there is no book or guidelines to advise me how to prescribe the drug? The professional associations of the medical doctors across Canada share my concerns.

I do not know what happens in the offices of primary care physicians, but I know what has happened at my clinic and other pain clinics since the decriminalization of pot for medical use. A number of patients have come forward asking for marijuana. Very few have their form signed by their family physician, but they make a formal request for a second opinion and approval, as it is required by law before they submit their application to the government. With the exception of the odd 75-year-old grandma with severe arthritis pain whose grandson will ask the question about pot use, in my estimation 90 per cent or more of those who have asked for medical use of pot so far from my clinic have been habitual pot smokers and users of all kinds of illegal drugs and booze before the onset of the condition for which they are referred to my clinic. The odd scruffy fellow will even wander into the clinic, obviously stoned, and ask the secretary, "Is she prescribing the stuff?" Only recently, I saw a 48-year-old woman with a drug-induced stroke and a horrendous history of intravenous drug abuse and multiple suicide attempts by overdose, who was sent to me by her family doctor with the question of medical marijuana use. She was the one to raise this issue—of course the poor family physician would not consider taking it upon his shoulders. Presumably she had tried every available drug and developed side effects with mini-doses. My alternative was to send her to a colleague for methadone—which would serve her much better for both her addictions and her pain.

I should note with some optimism that the federal government has recently granted sizable funding to researchers belonging to the Canadian Consortium on Cannabinoids, so that proper studies can be done on people. The consortium consists of medical doctors, other health care professionals and scientists. The studies are long overdue. While I am quite prepared to administer marijuana or synthetic cannabinoids in accepted forms other than smoking, I and many others need proper guidelines that are developed from well-designed trials. That is how medical knowledge advances, not by the hasty decisions of bureaucrats. For the time being, I am more than content recommending the proper use of the types of approved drugs I have information about, including opioids.

Nine

DO-IT-YOURSELF

Marcia, a college student, was referred to my clinic almost two years after the onset of bizarre swelling and pain in her right arm. She said that when she was 21, at work as a swim instructor with children, she experienced sudden pain shooting into her right elbow when she turned around quickly while her hand was resting on a table. Her elbow and hand swelled up within minutes. She visited a local emergency and this led to admission to the hospital, as the doctors were afraid that she had developed a clot in a deep vein and that this was obstructing the blood flow. But they could find no blood clot. Soon after, a bone scan showed abnormalities and a diagnosis of reflex sympathetic dystrophy (RSD) or complex regional pain syndrome was made.

RSD is a syndrome I have mentioned in this book. It occurs after an injury to an arm or a leg (many times it could be just a sprain), and is associated with terrific pain, swelling, hypersensitivity and changes in skin texture. The syndrome remains a major mystery for both clinicians and experimental scientists.

I have been involved in extensive research relating to RSD over many years, and in my own mind, all the symptoms and signs that Marcia reported can be seen in four types of situations. They can be the result of immobilization, fear of movement and complete avoidance of the use of a limb. They also occur sometimes in what we call "disease imitators"—in other words, in some cases disorders other than RSD account for the symptoms, such as tumours, inflammation or infection. A third type of situation is self-inflicted—some patients show up at the doctor with disorders they manufacture. Some, for example will squeeze or tie up the arm or the leg to generate visible signs of swelling, coldness and skin changes, so they can obtain money, drugs or attention. Finally, the symptoms that Marcia had could truly be attributed to what I call "real" RSD—when part of a patient's nervous system has been deranged. Unfortunately, the abnormalities in Marcia's bone scan were not easy for me to categorize, as they can occur in any or all of these situations.

Marcia went on carrying her arm in an unusual position for many months. She kept her swollen limb extended at the elbow and always hanging down, a bit like Popeye the Sailor. With some physical therapy, after nine months all signs disappeared and Marcia told me she was completely "normal." But that lasted only a month. She said that while watching a movie, she experienced similar problems with her left hand, though the problems disappeared within three days. These bizarre episodes—swelling or pain in the right or left arm that would appear and then subside out of the blue—continued. In January 2001, Marcia reported that her right arm swelled within 20 minutes while she was typing. From that time on, the swelling and pain never went away.

When I first saw her, several things were striking about Marcia's appearance. First, throughout the whole time she was with us, she kept her grotesquely deformed and swollen arm hanging down. Her hand was absurd looking; huge, puffy and spongy, like an inflated balloon. I had the feeling that her skin was going to burst open any time. Marcia sat in my office with a rather indifferent expression. She was unable to lift anything, bend or wiggle her fingers or move her elbow. Normally, such a grotesque deformity and a useless arm should be depressing for anyone, let alone a young woman. But Marcia did not seem distressed or depressed. As a matter of fact, she did not seem to care at all. It was as if this hand were not hers.

A careful inspection revealed clear rope-like marks around the elbow. When asked, Marcia told us she was using a tight bandage around the elbow to subdue the pain. It simply did not seem to occur to her, that choking her elbow while her arm hangs down immobile would strangle the limb and trap blood in the hand, leading to the severe swelling.

I doubted the diagnosis of RSD. My strong suspicion that this whole thing was simply manufactured was shared by my staff. I offered Marcia admission to the in-patient unit. I wanted very much to know what would happen to this stiff and unyielding arm of hers if I were to put her under a general anaesthetic. I was wondering whether Marcia's muscles had shrunk, given the fact she refused to move either her arm or her hand for many months. Had she permanently lost the range of movement in her joints, and if so, how much had she lost?

Amazingly, under general anaesthesia, her stiff immobile limb had complete and free range of movement in the shoulder, wrist and hand. Marcia had lost just a bit of range from the elbow, but nothing that could not be corrected by physiotherapy. So, when she woke up, we called the occupational therapist, who fabricated a special splint to hold Marcia's arm upward. The splint was fastened to an overhead trapeze bar. Within 12 hours the grotesque swelling decreased substantially.

Our team discussed her case extensively. We had no doubt that Marcia's bizarre swelling was just the result of immobility, her unusual posture and the tight bandage. The numbness and tingling she was complaining of in her fingers was nothing but the result of the swelling that choked the nerves. But what were the reasons behind the creation of such a monstrous arm? Could it be in her mind? Could it be related to Marcia's attitude toward her younger brother, who was "developmentally slow" with special needs? Perhaps deep down Marcia felt her brother had monopolized their parents' attention, and maybe Marcia's painful condition was a way of getting even. Or maybe it was even more complicated. Since Marcia planned to apply to the university to become a teacher for children with special needs, maybe somewhere in her mind she could believe that her "disability" could facilitate admission. Certainly, her behaviour and personality were unusual enough to make our conjectures plausible.

We did not confront Marcia directly with any of this. We simply indicated that probably the immobility and the dependent positioning of her arm were responsible for the swelling. We advised her to stop using the bandage to tie the elbow, and we made arrangements for home care visits, as well as outpatient occupational therapy to ensure that she was using the splint and elevating the arm. But things did not go as planned. The therapist approached me on several occasions to complain that Marcia would not listen to her. She would not wear the splint and would keep her arm hanging Popeye-style no matter what she was told.

In a subsequent visit, I had to be more forthright. "Listen," I said, "You do not comply with the treatment and you do not listen. You have to understand fully that unless you use the splint and avoid dependency of your arm, you are going to be in bigger trouble, maybe with blood clots and infection. All of us on the team consider you totally responsible for what is going on with your arm."

"Okay," she responded, showing no signs of upset or concern. She was so indifferent; it was as if I had been talking about someone else.

Soon after this confrontation, she hit her hand on a door knob. The X-rays showed a fractured right baby finger. The finger was taped tightly by her physician. Afterward, Marcia suddenly started wearing the splint we had made for her, for reasons that none of us understood. And of course, as we predicted, her hand shrunk soon after to a normal size.

Whatever bothered Marcia's hand was a "factitious" disease. Whether or not one is a doctor, the sight of such disfigurement makes one wonder: Why would Marcia do such things to herself? How often does a clinic like mine see patients of this sort? How far will these patients go in their expressions of disease? The answer to this last question is, "as far as one can possibly imagine."

Ronnie was referred to me in 1996 at the age of 44. His problems started a year before this referral, after an unusual accident that hurt his right middle finger. The wound did not seem to heal. He said that while he was working with some tools at home, he accidentally spilled hydrochloric acid on his right middle finger. This is a deadly poison that eats the flesh by burning it in short order. But, he added, when this happened he did not visit any doctor until four weeks later, when the pain became excruciating. As anyone would, I thought: How many of us would spill acid over our flesh and watch it rot away for weeks before we seek medical advice?

Eventually, Ronnie showed up at my hospital's emergency with a rotten and infected finger. He was admitted and treated with antibiotics. The surgeons wanted to amputate his finger immediately, as it had been literally eaten by the acid and the flesh was dead, but Ronnie refused. Several months later he gave in.

The amputation was carried out to the level of the first finger joint just below the knuckle. Normally the wound from an amputation will heal well as long as it is kept clean. But Ronnie's wound never healed. Despite the splints, the dressings and the antibiotics, the stump kept rotting away, while Ronnie complained bitterly of intractable pain. That's when he was referred to me.

He told me his pain was 9 out of 10, going all the way up to 15 out of 10 in bad situations, and opioids did not really help. Strangely, despite such high pain ratings, he did not seem to be in distress. He made sure we knew he was well off because of his job as an architect and a hefty inheritance. For a well-to-do architect, he looked rather scruffy, undernourished and generally ill. His clothes did not remind me of someone working in a prestigious job at a fancy office. When he took his shirt off for my examination, I was surprised to discover numerous scars all over his arms. I counted 14 in the left arm and 4 in the right. When I asked about the origin of one particularly deep and ugly scar that crossed almost the whole length of his right forearm, he said indifferently that a metal plate had accidentally torn his flesh at work. Needle tracks also checkered his arms. When he removed the right finger dressing, I panicked. The stump was charcoal black, a dead piece of mummified flesh with a ring of fresh tissue encircling the base of the amputated finger. This ring of pink flesh made me suspicious. I wondered whether the bone itself was infected under this necrotic stump. And of course, I wondered about a lot more. The bizarre components of Ronnie's story, the scars, the needle tracks, the architect who did not look like an architect, made me extremely suspicious.

We made several calls to his physicians. The same themes kept emerging—non-healing wounds for reasons not understood and too many requests for pain medications. Finally, we admitted Ronnie to our in-patient unit. By then, the black, dead skin had fallen off. The bone of the third finger was sticking out—grotesquely naked. There really was not a thread of flesh on it. Yet our tests failed to show any infection. So we concentrated on the man instead of the finger.

Extensive consultations with the psychiatrist and the psychologist added more fantastic detail to Ronnie's story, or more accurately, his stories. He told us he had gone through many surgeries to repair broken bones and nerve damage throughout his body. He said that one time he fell a great height from a ladder and broke his breastbone, the bones of his face, 17 ribs, both knees and "all the bones" at the top of his feet. Another time a steel plate went through his left hand, "requiring 11 operations." Just before the acid-spilling incident, he said he was trying to cut a piece of Plexiglas when he severed an artery and two nerves in his right hand. He provided considerable detail about the drugs he took for pain, specifying some strong narcotics that "he could not do without."

His personal history was similarly convoluted and grandiose. Ronnie said that Canada's well-known astronaut Roberta Bondar was his half-sister. He also said that he had graduated from the University of Toronto in 1979 after a four-year architectural drafting program. But he could not remember any of his professors' names and he appeared to have little knowledge of his profession. He said he had a son who was a dentist and that an uncle had died some years ago, leaving him millions. To top this, Ronnie claimed that he had designed some of Toronto's most celebrated buildings. Predictably, when we called his wife, she said Ronnie was no architect, Roberta Bondar was not his sister, they had no son and there was no inheritance.

Detailed psychological tests and consultations with the psychiatry department all pointed to an unusual degree of psychopathology. Our team concluded that Ronnie's wound was self-inflicted, to obtain drugs and attention. The grandiose and false information Ronnie provided made us concerned about a delusional disorder. We felt that the way he was going, he could do even more serious harm to himself. We strongly suggested admission to a psychiatric institution adjacent to our facilities, but not only did Ronnie refuse, he discharged himself before we were able to make any arrangements. We could do little other than to communicate the information we had gathered to Ronnie's physician, so the doctor could try to persuade Ronnie to accept admission for psychiatric treatment.

Jackie was 31 when she leaned on her husband's weight-lifting bench and some of the heavy weight plates fell, crushing her left forearm. Her arm swelled up like a soap bubble. She needed emergency surgery to release the tight and swollen muscles, but her pain continued unabated. She was checked afterward for possible clots in her veins, but none were found. Because her pain was not improving, the surgeons opened up her forearm again, searching for trapped nerves, but in vain. She also had several nerve blocks at the web of the neck to try to soothe the pain, but they did not work either. She was finally referred to us with the possible diagnosis of RSD.

When seen in my clinic by Tea, one of the younger physicians on our team, Jackie complained of constant, sharp, burning and stinging pain in her afflicted forearm. As usually happens with neuropathic pains, a simple touch, a cold draft or the slightest movements would aggravate her. She was taking a fair amount of opioids and several combinations of antidepressants and medications for anxiety. Since the accident, Jackie, a mother of two children under 10, had stopped working as a radiology technician and needed considerable help from her husband to take a bath, dress and get in and out of her car.

After taking the history, Tea walked out of her office and called me to see Jackie. She was puzzled. "I know she had several surgeries and her forearm is scarred all over. But something is strange," she said.

"Her forearm is dark red, extremely sensitive to touch and looks awful. She does not allow me to get close to it. But, forgive me for being suspicious; I thought I saw some red powder on her beige pants. The colour of the powder is similar to the red of her forearm."

We both wondered what to do. I came up with a plan. "Just say you are calling the director of the program to take a look at her because her condition is complex," I told Tea.

I entered the examining room holding a Kleenex soaked in water behind my back. Jackie warned me she was intolerant to touch. As I introduced myself, I took a swipe at her forearm without asking her or giving her any warning. "What are you doing?" she yelled and withdrew her arm abruptly. Bingo! There it was, a purple-red stain on my tissue, leaving a long clean strip of skin where I had wiped Jackie's arm. Whatever I had wiped off looked like reddish makeup. The skin seemed normal where the paint had come off. Jackie stood there dumbfounded. She did not say anything, but within seconds she knew it was time—no pun intended—to come clean.

"Jackie, are you painting your arm?" I asked.

"Yes," she admitted hesitantly. "The skin is so bad that I wanted to make it look more natural."

I pointed to the clean strip of flesh. "Jackie, this is clean and normal skin. It looks just fine. It is the rest of your forearm all painted purplish that is so unnatural and attracts attention." From that point on the examination went downhill quickly. Jackie refused to move her arm or hand, saying it was too painful to do so. We could not even touch her to check deep tendon reflexes with our little hammer.

When we offered Jackie admission to our in-patient unit, she refused. She left surrounded by several men, her husband, brother and friends, all attentive and, I thought, overprotective.

Why would this woman engage in such a deception? Without question she had sustained a crushing injury, and the first surgery to release the tightness in her arm was justified. But what about all the other surgeries, investigations and injections? They were all performed because of intractable pain, but yielded no good results. So what was the real problem? This formerly independent working mother had now become a highly dependent individual, needing help even for her personal hygiene. Maybe her relationship with her husband had something to do with it. Maybe he felt guilty for her injury in his gym and maybe his care and attentiveness were what Jackie liked the most and she would do everything she could to maintain—including painting her arm.

Jackie, Ronnie and Marcia all had one thing in common: they themselves were responsible for creating the ailment that brought them to the doctors. In all cases something had gone physically wrong in the first place, but subsequently it was the patients who would do everything they could to sustain and magnify the problem. Their cases fall under the medical term of "factitious disorder" (self-induced afflictions).

Factitious disorders form a spectrum of abnormal illness behaviours. The best-known form, Munchausen's syndrome, was first described by a British neurologist in 1951.[1] The syndrome was named after Baron Karl Friedrich Hieronymus von Munchausen, a war hero in the eighteenth-century German cavalry. He became famous for telling stories about himself, full of impressive and unbelievable events. Usually such patients have one or more dramatic but factitious (self-induced) complaints. They lie extensively and use multiple medical and other services, going from hospital to hospital and from city to city. It is their incredible fabrications and distortions of their true histories that led to the use of Munchausen's name to label the syndrome.

Munchausen's can also be extrapolated from a parent to a child. In such cases it is known as Munchausen's syndrome by proxy. This version of the syndrome has been made the theme of TV and large-screen movies (although the 1989 movie *The Adventures of Baron Munchausen* was not about Munchausen's syndrome or the proxy version). Munchausen's by proxy is created by a parent or a caregiver who produces a factitious disorder in a child. Studies show that while factitious disorders rarely result in death, Munchausen's by proxy can result in the death of the child victim.[2]

Diagnosing and understanding factitious disorders takes a lot of work by the physician, who has to take into account the patient's personal history, causes of personal stress and family dynamics. Beneath the surface of many factitious disorders lies a disturbed, unstable personality—one that subconsciously seeks attention by assuming the role of the sick person. Often, an acute loss—of a spouse or another loved one, or of a house or job—seems to precipitate Munchausen's syndrome and other factitious disorders.

Another type of factitious disorder is Ganser's syndrome, which was first described in the nineteenth century by a German psychiatrist, who observed prisoners attempting to avoid unpleasant events or obtain sick privileges. In this syndrome, patients simulate madness and produce unusual or irrational answers to simple questions like, "How many legs does a cow have?" Such a patient may answer, "Three!" Ganser's syndrome differs from Munchausen's in that in cases of Ganser's, the behaviours are both conscious (for example, to avoid work) and subconscious, while in Munchausen's syndrome the gains are a subconscious bid to gain attention.

Malingering is another form of manufactured disorder. This is when a person simulates a disease or symptom for obvious gains like money or drugs. But in cases of malingerers, the reasons are clear and not subconscious, as in Munchausen's syndrome. Unfortunately, research shows that neither lay people nor professionals such as psychologists, doctors and lawyers are good at identifying liars and embellishers. Malingering usually cannot be determined in a single interview. It is actually quite inappropriate for a professional to make such a diagnosis unless there is unequivocal collateral information from reliable sources. There is an added disincentive in making such a diagnosis in that a professional who does so risks being sued or punished.

An example that hits rather close to home for me is what happened to a well-known Ontario neuropsychologist, Dr. Frank Kenny. I know Frank well, as his office was close to mine during the start of my career. After a thorough assessment of a claimant on behalf of a large car insurance company, including the administration of special tests that can show if one fabricates his or her symptoms, Frank concluded that this person "was consciously feigning his problems for personal gain." The claimant's lawyer complained to the Ontario College of Psychologists, which laid charges against Dr. Kenny. The legal battles took many years. Although there was no doubt that the claimant was indeed fabricating his symptoms, the College found Dr. Kenny guilty for using some spurious words and applied a small penalty. But Dr. Kenny refused to accept it. He appealed the charges to the Divisional Court of Ontario. Hundreds of thousands of dollars and years later, the court unanimously struck down the decision of the Ontario College of Psychologists, and ordered the College to pay all costs from the very beginning of Dr. Kenny's ordeal. Frank was vindicated, but after years of legal wrangling, his practice had disintegrated and his personal costs were enormous. His case sent a clear message to practising psychologists that the diagnosis of malingering would at best be ill-advised and at worst would reap unfortunate consequences, even when justified.

In medico-legal cases, for example when injuries are sustained in a car accident, allegations of malingering are not infrequent. But one must be careful and have unequivocal proof of symptom feigning before the diagnosis is made. This unequivocal proof may be difficult to obtain. About 10 years ago, I was asked to examine someone in a case that shows how far one must sometimes go to get decisive proof of malingering. Juan, a man in his early 30s from Ecuador, had been involved in a minor car accident, a fender-bender. But at the scene of the accident, he was unable to get out of the car. The ambulance took him to one of the trauma centres in Toronto on a stretcher. Juan never moved his legs since the accident, and for all intents and purposes he had become a paraplegic. But the doctors could never put a picture together of what exactly was wrong. Juan insisted he had no feeling and no power in his legs, but his reflexes were still there. Moreover, his legs did not waste away, which is what happens in cases of damaged nerves or spinal cord injury, and his bladder was in perfect shape—also something that is unusual for paraplegics. Spinal CAT scans and MRIs failed to show any abnormality in the spinal cord. Juan was hospitalized in a spinal cord injury rehabilitation unit and was taught how to use his wheelchair and how to transfer from the chair to the car or the bathtub.

He was referred to me by his auto insurer for an examination: the company was concerned because if his condition were permanent, it would have to pick up millions of dollars of living and medical costs for the rest of Juan's life. When there is a tough, complicated case like this, my unit is often asked to investigate thoroughly, to tease out the biomedical versus the psychological components of pain. There were only two possible diagnoses in Juan's case: hysteria, also known as conversion reaction (in which bizarre neurological symptoms are the physical expressions of disturbed emotions), or plain, ordinary malingering and symptom fabrication. I offered admission to Juan. "No problem, Doctor," he said. "I would love to get better."

"Good, it's a deal. You will be with us for five days and will be discharged on Friday," I told him.

"But I will leave at 6 o'clock every night to go home and then come back in the morning, right?"

"Absolutely wrong, Juan. You stay in the hospital for the duration of the investigations—day and night until all our work is completed."

There was a reason for my insistence. I wanted a patient like Juan to be observed on the ward by nurses and other hospital staff, who could detect and document his pain behaviours, interactions with other patients, his transfers from chair to bed, his sleeping positions and so on. Unfortunately, Juan, feeling he was heading toward dangerous ground, refused admission. I suspected that malingering was the most likely diagnosis, but I could not really say more, as I had no definite proof.

From that time on, his insurer went on a spending spree. They hired private investigators who collected extensive film footage and videotape of Juan—recording him leaving his house (always with a young female companion whom he called his assistant), going to the market, wheeling his chair in the park, getting in and out of the car, all this over many months. Finally, the insurance company came back to me with several tapes to watch. After months of taping and many thousands of dollars, the insurers felt they had unquestionable proof of his ability to walk in footage of approximately 60 decisive seconds, and they wanted me to identify Juan in the tape.

How the investigators managed to shoot this remarkable minute that made Juan's carefully orchestrated paralysis act, perfected over many years, fall to pieces, I do not know. The videographer must have had wings to be able to shoot some of the footage. The tape showed Juan rolling his wheelchair in front of the door to his home. His female companion opened the door for him to get in and closed it behind him. A minute or two later a male figure went into what seemed to be the bathroom. The blinds were only half turned, so he could be easily seen. Seconds later, that figure got up and walked to the sink to wash his face. I was sure it was Juan—I could tell by the colour of his hair and the red shirt that he was wearing when he wheeled up to the door and when he walked to the bathroom sink.

After years of deception, Juan was caught. Later it turned out that Juan had been defrauding the welfare system as well, as he had managed to collect payments from both the car insurance company and the provincial government. Was Juan "normal" in terms of personality? I seriously doubt it. Anyone who can remain for several years in a wheelchair whenever he leaves the house could not possibly be healthy, even if financial gain was a motive for doing this. Juan's case demonstrated to me conclusively that malingering is just a part of a spectrum of abnormal illness behaviours.

No one really knows how often self-induced disorders occur. It is generally presumed that they are exceedingly rare. But at clinics like mine, which see the hardest and most puzzling cases, the statistics may be different. We did a study over a two-year period recently in our clinic to find out how many patients we saw every year who were like Ronnie, Marcia and Jackie, with visible and grotesque physical abnormalities, that we proved beyond doubt to be self-inflicted. We only came up with something like 1 to 2 per cent of all our new patient consultations. However, when we looked only at those referred to us as possible reflex sympathetic dystrophy (RSD) cases, the figures increased to about 8 per cent. There are many reasons for this. The symptoms of true RSD are by their nature difficult to understand, as they are many and variable.

Several of them can be easily reproduced by immobility or by tying up the limb and fooling the untrained eye. Unfortunately, in none of the cases referred to us that were as obvious as those of Marcia and Jackie did the physicians who referred the patients ever suspect factitious disorders.

Many examples demonstrate the magnitude of symptom fabrication (and of course chronic pain is claimed to be a major problem in these cases), particularly in motor vehicle cases. Tort claims have become a political issue. In 1988, the Southeastern Pennsylvania Transportation Authority (SEPTA) initiated a Fraudulent Claims Program, trying to look more closely at the U.S.$53 million the state makes in yearly payments for about 15,000 personal injury claims. The FBI got involved in investigating suspicious claims. For example, in one serious public transit accident, seven passengers filed claims for injuries sustained in the crash, but only one passenger was found to be in the vehicle at the time of the accident. The other six allegedly injured passengers were indicted for fraud by a grand jury.[3] A 73-year-old doctor was sentenced to 15 months in jail and fined U.S.$100,000 for providing false testimony.[4] Once it became known that SEPTA was after cheaters, injury claims against the authority fell by 60 per cent and lawsuits by 50 per cent, resulting in multimillion-dollar savings for the financially strapped transit agency.[5]

One small New Jersey bus company was plagued by injury claims for fender-bender type accidents. The company asked the New Jersey Insurance Fraud Division to investigate, and in "Operation Bus Roulette," the fraud division staged 10 minor bus accidents throughout New Jersey.[6] They were all video-taped and Connie Chung, then with CBS, participated in one of the crashes with her *Eye To Eye* team. The *Eye To Eye* "Undercover Report" was aired in August 1992 and showed 17 people who had been walking by the crash site enter the bus *after* the accident.[7] All 17 later submitted claims for injuries, ranging from U.S.$30,000 to $400,000 per claim. Operation Bus Roulette caught more than 100 people ripping off insurance companies, including 10 doctors and 4 lawyers.[8]

There are many examples of the magnitude of fraud where I live, too. In the summer of 2000, the Toronto police launched "Project Slip," charging 35 people, including 5 physicians, in a multimillion-dollar insurance scam for staged car accidents and tumbles in buses and streetcars.[9] In another instance, after a staged accident with a rental car, the police launched Canada's biggest auto insurance fraud investigation ever. The search discovered a large Toronto auto insurance fraud ring, responsible for 257 suspicious claims worth $10 million and relating to more than 60 staged car accidents. Fifty-four people were involved, including physicians and chiropractors.[10]

When I contemplate the lack of training we physicians get to distinguish real patients from those who feign problems, as well as the fact that we "do not see what we are not looking for," I am sure I have missed more fakers than the ones I have caught. But it's important to note that not all self-afflicted disorders are factitious.

Biting the Hand That Hurts

Jim was sitting across from me. He was slender, bearded, in his 30s, his shirt open to mid-chest, his nose slightly crooked—perhaps as a testimony to an old fistfight—definitely good-looking. But he had a hard time answering my questions.

I was delving into the details of his pain: when did it start, what part of the body it covered, did it change during the day and so on. He did not seem to pay much attention to me, as he was preoccupied, biting his fingers, viciously gnawing at the right hand that was giving him so much pain.

Almost two years earlier, Jim had taken a tumble down several stairs after drinking a few beers, and had gotten himself into some serious trouble. He suffered a mild head injury and managed to pull some of the roots of his right brachial plexus, the bundle of nerves responsible for the sensation and the movements of his arm. He also damaged a nerve in his right leg. He described his pains as burning, tingling, pricking, stinging and freezing. He could not tolerate simple touching or gentle pricking with a needle over the arm and hand. He had a hard time wearing his shoe on the foot of his injured leg. But his hand was the worst: he could not stop chewing constantly on that same very painful, deformed and clawed appendage, day and night. Mary, his girlfriend, told me that he often woke up with his hand and lips soaked in blood. At times, too, he would bang his painful leg forcefully against the wall.

"Jim," I said, watching him as he munched on his fingers, "Why, for God's sake, do you do this?"

He answered quickly. "I hate this hand. Can't you see how ugly it is? It makes me want to cry. Sometimes the pain is so strong that I feel like chopping the hand and the leg off. I don't seem to be able to stop. It's as if something inside me pushes me to chew the fingers, even if it makes me hurt more!"

Jim's case was similar to that of another patient of mine, Simon. He developed RSD in the first two fingers of his left hand and ended up scratching them to the point of bleeding every time he got painful itching spells. Later, he started rubbing his hand with a hand-held vibrator with a rubber tip. Then he progressed to a razor blade, literally skinning off the fingers, even though he was creating more pain. I ended up putting his hand in a cast to protect it. Simon admitted that he was unable to stop hurting himself; the urge was beyond his control. As all this evolved, Simon became profoundly depressed and his marriage fell apart.

Jim and Simon had several things in common. Both had suffered a partial injury or dysfunction of the nervous system that produced pain, and each of them had an uncontrollable urge to attack the painful limb. Both were angry and depressed. All these are characteristic of a larger behaviour pattern. This is self-injurious behaviour—attacking the part that hurts.

I had seen a few other cases in my life like Simon and Jim and had kept a little blue diary with their names and conditions. Every time I come across such patients, I find it truly unbelievable to see people with normal intelligence attacking parts of their body and admitting to it. They knew they were hurting and harming their bodies more, but they could not resist the urge to attack, driven by incessant pain. The behaviour of these patients is strikingly different from that of a malingerer or those with Munchausen's syndrome, who deny that they create the symptoms and signs themselves.

Similar self-injurious behaviours are observed in laboratory animals after injury to the nerves of a limb. In scientific terms the phenomenon is called autotomy (from the Greek words *auto*, meaning "self," and *tomi*, meaning "cutting"). Injured rats and monkeys autotomize themselves by scratching, mutilating or even self-cannibalizing the "denervated" part. This type of behaviour had been attributed by many laboratory scientists to pain produced by the nerve injury.

Some researchers thought that it is pain that compels desperate animals to get rid of this aching yet insensitive limb. Other scientists, however, fervently disputed this idea, believing that the animals bite away an insensitive limb just to get rid of a useless appendage, the way a lizard sheds away the old, useless tail. Because animals don't talk, the debate went on and on. As scientists continued to debate why the animals were autotomizing themselves, published reports of human beings attacking a painful body part were extremely rare.

So I decided to search the literature. First, I found out that self-injurious behaviour has been reported quite often in humans who do not have pain. It is a dramatic but poorly understood phenomenon. Common forms of this behaviour include cutting and burning the skin, banging the head and other body parts, picking at wounds and chewing fingers. At times the injuries can be severe—some people go so far as to amputate their own tongues or fingers, or to create wounds that don't heal and become infected. This behaviour has been seen in individuals with serious mental retardation, in patients with psychosis and other mental illnesses, and among prisoners who have been provoked or aggravated by stress and isolation.[11]

Researchers have focused on the biological aspects of this self-injurious behaviour. In experiments with animals, abnormalities have been reported in internal (endogenous) analgesic systems working through opioids, dopamine and serotonin. Studies in humans have also raised the suspicion of neurotransmitter abnormalities. The human studies in particular have connected violent and impulsive behaviour toward one's own body (and against others) with abnormal serotoninergic function.[12]

I knew nothing about these phenomena in people, until the cases of Jim, Simon and two other patients of mine made their way to my little blue book. As I continued my search through seemingly endless literature, I discovered to my surprise that there were numerous cases of patients reported to hurt themselves the way Simon and Jim did. All these patients had some injury to the peripheral nerves or the central nervous system—injuries such as neuralgia, neuropathy, spinal cord injury, brachial plexus avulsion, certain types of stroke and intracranial tumours. But the majority of the cases were related to damage of the trigeminal nerve after alcohol injections or root surgery. The trigeminal nerve primarily supplies sensation to the face, jaw and mouth.

As discussed earlier, the unfortunate sufferers of trigeminal neuralgia experience short bouts of excruciating sharp, knife-like pains, triggered by chewing, yawning, a mere touch or other simple stimuli to certain parts of the face. Neurosurgeons try to make this nerve unresponsive by injecting nerve-killing alcohol or other nerve-killing chemicals, such as phenol or glycerol, or through surgery. Some unlucky patients, particularly after alcohol injection in the nerve, will rid themselves of the original pain and replace it with a new pain consisting of very unpleasant sensations called dysesthesiae. The new disorder that appears combines a totally insensitive skin area with painful sensations underneath the skin and is called anaesthesia dolorosa. Patients provide us with vivid descriptions of the painful sensations—a "deep gnawing," feeling "as if the side of my face is on fire" or "feeling like my skin has been invaded by ants."[13] Some of these patients persistently and compulsively attack the anaesthesized but painful side of the face. However, when the pain is managed successfully with drugs, electrical stimulation or surgery, the behaviour ceases.

After my own search, I published a paper in the journal of the International Association for the Study of Pain in 1996, in which I presented my four cases and reviewed others.[14] I concluded that this behaviour occurs in a few patients with peripheral or central nervous system damage, who exclusively attack the painful part. Usually this part seems to be insensitive to pain, but in rare cases it may be hypersensitive. The behaviour is compulsive and uncontrollable, which the patients admit. It seems to be triggered or facilitated by boredom, isolation, depression, frustration, drug abuse, abnormal personality and occasionally pre-existing habits, like nail biting. I felt that these attacks to the painful body part are "released" or "facilitated" by a combination of genetic, personality, hormonal/neurohumeral and environmental factors in the presence of peripheral or central nervous system lesions. In this respect, I proposed that humans actually do resemble the animals who "autotomize" themselves. It seems that my patients were able to answer the question the animals could not: yes, the limb is attacked because it hurts. This paper has been quoted frequently in the international literature on the subject, so it seems that the phenomenon of animal autotomy is finally gaining acceptance as an indication of intractable neuropathic pain.

I was learning something slowly. It does not matter how advanced we humans think we are, the biological and behavioural similarities between us and animals as small as rats and as big and developed as monkeys can be stunning.

I lost Jim from my care after a couple of years. Later, I found out he was residing in a jail cell. His impulsive nature, his poor judgment and his alcohol and drug abuse took their toll. Simon, on the other hand, has been with me many years. The stresses in his life are still so serious that I think they are the stuff movies are made of. But once his extremely painful, itchy spells decreased on their own, his attacks to his hand were much less frequent, even if his life remains terrible.

I think I am right that in these cases, this behaviour is not brought on by just one factor, such as depression. For such behaviours to happen, you need the biology to go wrong too, you need the marriage of the physical injury with the psychology and distorted feelings.

Clearly these cases support my view of looking at pain from a "whole person perspective."

Ten

MIND GAMES

An Arm and a Leg

I met Daniel in 1993, when he was 34. Before the injury that led him to my clinic, he was working as a truck driver, bringing home $125,000 a year. He was an athletic, multitalented man, involved in martial arts and a diehard biker. But when he injured his back at work, things changed for him dramatically. His doctors found a large herniated disc compressing one of his nerve roots and generating pain in his back and left leg. They operated and removed a disc with a procedure called microdiscectomy, performed with the help of a tiny tube inserted into his spine through a small incision in his back. Things seemed to improve with physiotherapy until some weeks into his recovery, when Daniel twisted his back accidentally. Pain returned with a vengeance in his back and his left leg, but this time things were different. When he saw me, I knew that something was very strange.

Daniel had no sensation at all in the left leg, the one that hurt him deeply. "Look doctor," he would say, "I feel nothing," as he smacked the leg with his wooden cane, to the point where he was bruising it. He went on: "The floor feels funny under my foot, as though I'm walking on feathers." His right arm was painful too. He had hurt it as well during the work accident. Amazingly, this arm had no sensation either, from the elbow to his fingers.

Sensation can be skin sensation (a sharp pinprick, the touch of a tissue or something cold) or deep sensation (pressure, the movement of a body part or vibration). Daniel had lost all forms of sensation in these two painful limbs. Puzzled because I had never seen this before, I put him through many tests. I could find nothing wrong with his arm. When it came to his leg, CAT scans and MRIs of the lumbar spine did show some scarring around the left fifth lumbar nerve root (nerve root fibrosis). But this scarring could in no way explain the abrupt and complete loss of sensation in the whole leg, starting just below the groin level. It was as if somebody had drawn a straight line with a marker. Daniel had been told that since his sensory loss could not be explained by any tests, his pain was in his head. Understandably, this had upset him very much.

I admitted Daniel to my in-patient unit. I was going to test him with a special drug called sodium amytal. It belongs to the barbiturate family and has been used since the First World War on patients with serious emotional traumas to help them relax and open up both their consciousness and their hearts. Such emotionally traumatized persons could arrive for treatment mute, deaf or having lost their memory. Amytal would then somehow open up their brain and "probe their unconscious," digging out fears and emotional traumas, thus helping them to recover their memory, their hearing or their ability to talk. Because of these unique properties, the drug has also become popularly known—particularly for those who read mysteries or comic books—as "truth serum."

Sometime during the mid-1980s, I had made the accidental observation that intravenous sodium amytal produced dramatic and unexpected effects on a patient who had a damaged nerve in his right foot. The drug's action in this man proved to be quite different from those "mind-relaxing" effects described above. Within minutes, my patient's cold, blue foot turned hot and pink, while all abnormal sensitivity to the touch (allodynia) disappeared. After this unbelievable observation, my team did a fair amount of research, administering intravenous sodium amytal and confirming the drug's amazing actions in discriminating neuropathic from nociceptive pains. We published our findings and for many years since, the drug has been a standard tool in my armoury for teasing out the different mechanisms that can underlay pain.[1]

When I tested Daniel with the drug in 1994, something unusual happened: His pain started dropping fast, as the amytal was going into his bloodstream. It dropped from an 8 out of 10 to a 3 in his left leg and from a 6 to 1 in his right arm. This effect was not unusual—it is seen often in many patients with chronic pain who have been tested with the drug. What is startling and unusual (in fact, something I had never seen before) was that the sensation started returning to Daniel's anaesthetic limbs. As his pain was shrinking, Daniel was rediscovering the touch and the prickly feeling that he had lost for so many years. He was shedding his anaesthesia as if he were removing a stocking slowly from the groin to the foot and a glove from the elbow to the fingers. I videotaped him (something I do with all my in-patients after they sign an informed consent). I have since played this tape at many scientific gatherings, as it shows Daniel's amazing reaction to the drug far more clearly than thousands of descriptive words ever could. On tape, Daniel tested himself with the pinwheel, squeezed his leg and finally stamped his foot on the floor, discovering with delight that he now could "feel" the wooden planks under his bare sole. "Dr. Mailis," he said ecstatically, "If I can stay like this, I swear I will walk on Yonge Street [a major street in Toronto] with my head down and my feet up!"

Unfortunately, the effect lasted only five to six hours and then the anaesthesia and the pain returned.

I tested Daniel again over the years at least five times. I often tried to trick him by giving him plain sterile water (normal saline) before or after the amytal, or I coloured the saline infusion with vitamins to make it look like a different drug. Even my staff played tricks on me (in the interest of investigation) by exchanging the order of normal saline and amytal without me knowing. No matter what we did, Daniel's pain and anaesthesia would invariably shrink only under the influence of amytal, and only for a few hours. I had put Daniel repeatedly through all kinds of tests and except for the little scarring in his left fifth lumbar root, all the wiring in his nervous system was intact.

I had no scientific explanation for the complete loss of sensation. Daniel came to my office regularly every three months so I could check him and document the levels of pain and loss of sensation in his left leg and right arm.

During one such visit, Daniel brought me unexpected news: "Dr. Mailis, you won't believe it but the feeling came back in my right arm and the pain is all gone." Indeed, as I tested him, I confirmed that the sensation was back in the arm, while the pain he had been feeling constantly had disappeared. This was now an absolutely normal arm with fluid movements and normal sensitivity to pinching and pressure, and it was free of any bizarre deep pain or skin pain. No specific reason, no particular event in Daniel's life could account for this, and for the life of me, I had no idea whatsoever what was going on.

But six or seven months later, the sensation again disappeared from Daniel's arm, in the same mysterious way it had recovered. "I cannot even describe to you what happened to me, because it sounds crazy," Daniel said. He went on to tell me a story that any sane person would have a hard time believing. Daniel was the back-seat passenger in the family car, with his wife driving and his young son sitting in the front. When he got out of the car and closed the door behind him, he realized he could not move much; it was as if something were gluing him to the vehicle. "Can't you see?" his wife yelled. Daniel turned behind, just to realize that the door had closed on his hand. He had no sensation and no idea whatsoever what had happened to his arm or where the arm was. From that time to this date, many years later, Daniel still has an anaesthetic right arm (from the elbow to the fingers) but luckily, he has no spontaneous pain whatsoever. The leg story, however, is different, as the pain continues to be persistent and bizarre.

By the time Daniel came and told me about the car door incident, I had become convinced that whatever was blocking his sensation had to be in his brain, and had to be temporary, coming and going but definitely not fixed or permanently damaged. So I went to a friend, Dr. Karen Davis, a researcher in the same hospital as my clinic, who specializes in the study of awake and thinking brains with a magnetic resonance imaging (MRI) machine. This type of MRI study is called "functional" MRI (fMRI), as the activity that is picked up corresponds to the energy consumption of activated brain cells. This is a research tool, not the typical everyday MRI that is used to look for herniated discs or tumours. When we tested Daniel the results were astounding. "His somatosensory cortex [the right part of the brain that corresponds to the left leg] is not responding normally," Karen said. Daniel's brain was properly activated when stimuli were applied to his healthy right leg. But when the stimuli were applied to his anaesthetic leg, sometimes his brain did not react at all and sometimes it became suppressed. In other words, when Daniel would say, "I do not feel," he really meant it, as his brain was not picking up whatever was going on in his leg.

"We cannot present these results anywhere, Angela," Karen said. "Our fMRI machine is so old and outdated that people will believe this is just a technical error." So Daniel's fMRI results were stored out of sight and forgotten by everyone . . . except me.

Strange Arms and Legs

Daniel's case opened windows in my own mind. I became more vigilant, looking more carefully at my patients. As my research progressed, it became obvious that phenomena like Daniel's bizarre pains in limbs that were otherwise literally senseless occurred quite frequently in patients who came to my clinic. Depending on the patient, the loss of sensation would vary from mild to intense. Our team's psychologist, Dr. Keith Nicholson, and I named these sensory abnormalities "non-dermatomal somatosensory deficits." This term was chosen to stress that the loss-of-sensation patterns were not following known territories of nerve or nerve root innervation of the skin. I reviewed the literature to find out who else had reported these phenomena and what scientists think of them. It turned out that these sensory deficits had actually been described for hundreds of years. Given the fact they were bizarre and could not be explained by injury to a given nerve or nerve root, the most common belief was that they were "psychogenic," "hysterical," or "non-organic." Such words mean that the loss of sensation is the product of thoughts or psychological disturbances alone, with no physical basis—something that is all in your head.

I found only two modern scientific studies that described these deficits in patients with chronic pain. Among almost 250 patients attending a chronic

Even more interesting was the fact that 75 per cent of those with these sensory deficits were born in countries other than Canada, compared with 57 per cent in the group without the sensory deficits. Did this mean that our country of birth and our cultural background influence the appearance of these bizarre deficits? The thought was provocative (and politically incorrect), so I felt I had to thoroughly check the actual data. My suspicion was confirmed. The majority of patients in the group with the sensory abnormalities were born in Southern Europe. Since I was convinced that these sensory deficits had their origin in the brain, such data meant that perhaps culture might also play a role in the way our brains react to an emotional or physical trauma. Since multiple studies in the clinic and the laboratory have shown that culture profoundly affects our reaction to and expression of pain, maybe the thought that culture too affects the very way our nervous system is wired was not far-fetched. All the patients in the group with the sensory deficits displayed intense pain behaviours and, without exception, they were all unemployed. By comparison, 31 per cent of the patients in the other group were back in the workforce. Without doubt something was special about the patients who had sensory deficits, persistent severe pain and high levels of disability without any serious detectable pathology.

A remarkable and extreme case was Francesca, whom we reported in our publication. She was born in Portugal and had come to Canada at the age of 20. When she was 37, she was involved in a rather insignificant car accident. She was driving, wearing her seat belt, when somebody hit her car from behind. Francesca's mind went immediately "blank" as she thought she "was going to die." Instantly, she felt "total body pain," her left side worse than her right, and became nearly paralyzed. She was taken to a local emergency and was let go the same day, as nothing was broken. By the time she arrived at my door two and a half years later, she had gone through all kinds of therapies—physiotherapy, chiropractic treatments, acupuncture, aquatherapy and so on. She had also tried handfuls of different medications, none of which helped. Several tests failed to find any good cause for her diffuse debilitating pains. She was bedridden, housebound and dependent on her husband for basic tasks. When I saw her, she gave me an endless list of complaints about every part of her body. She managed to draw her pains on a diagram, marking the left side of the body as the worst one. It would be hard to forget the sight of Francesca's appearance in my office. She walked stooped over, supported by her husband or clinging to walls, leaning on chairs, moaning and groaning and dragging her left leg, while she held her left arm tightly to her chest. If I did not know why she was coming to see me, I would swear she had suffered a stroke. During the visit, she looked spaced out, face expressionless, voice soft. However, on a couple of occasions she cried. Large blisters covered her left forearm. When I asked, I was told she had just burned herself two weeks before, attempting to take something out of the oven—but she did not feel it. As it turned out, Francesca had a complete loss of sensation, both on her skin and deeper, throughout the whole left side of her body. The same side that was so painful looked as if it were partially paralyzed.

As I had predicted, based on my experience with several such patients, during sodium amytal testing she nearly lost her anaesthesia from the left side of her body at the same time that she experienced pain relief. The team psychologist and psychiatrist saw her as part of our multidisciplinary team approach. We concluded that there was a substantial psychological element contributing to Francesca's pain and disability. The fabric of her personality was such that she tended to convert emotional conflicts into somatic symptoms. We thought that given Francesca's personality, the combination of an acute physical trauma (sprained and bruised muscles) and emotional trauma (she perceived the accident as life-threatening) was capable of generating a chain of reactions between her brain and her body. As all physical treatments alone had failed, we strongly recommended a cognitive-behavioural program combined with physical restoration and an exploration of her family dynamics, considering her tremendous dependence on an overprotective husband.

I was convinced that the appearance of these sensory deficits was a sign that Francesca's recovery was going to be difficult. Based on our experience with such patients we knew that once the sensory abnormalities showed up, the pain would become intractable and difficult to manage. With Dr. Nicholson, we attributed these deficits to "altered brain processing"—changes in the way the brain was reacting to a physically and emotionally traumatic event. We felt strongly that researchers should look further in exploring the neurological circuits responsible for these sensory deficits, as well as looking at the role of personality or stressful life events in the appearance of these abnormalities.

The story became extremely interesting and challenging. For years, doctors had taken these unexplained deficits as a sign of "non-organic" pain. But what is "organic" pain in the first place? I suppose it means pain coming from a body part where there is anatomical (structural) damage in muscles, tendons, bones or nervous tissue. When doctors order tests to detect abnormalities, the tests they order depend on what they think the origin of the problem might be. More often than not, damage in bones and joints can be shown with X-rays or bone scans. Electrophysiological techniques such as electromyographic and nerve conduction studies or somatosensory evoked potentials test the integrity of the peripheral nerves or the overall neural wiring from the limbs to the brain. Lesions to the spinal cord and brain are investigated with radiological techniques such as computerized axonic tomography (CAT scans) and magnetic resonance imaging (MRIs). When the results from all these tests are normal, whatever the patient suffers from is usually labelled "non-organic," and more often than not, it is assumed that whatever is wrong must be in the patient's head.

Our work was showing exactly this. Whatever was wrong with patients like Daniel and Francesca truly was in their heads—their brains, to be precise. Certainly it was not anatomical or structural, as all the tests were coming up as normal or showing only a small problem. Besides, if these sensory deficits were permanent, I would not be able to remove them for a few hours with amytal. Since all patients are not the same (some have some physical problems that I could find, some others do not), I had to try to understand who was going to develop these abnormalities under what circumstances.

As I was venturing now into the realm of brain, mind and emotions, I was embarking into unknown waters—the murky sea where the body and the mind encounter each other and interact, sometimes in bizarre and incomprehensible ways. To my way of thinking, emotions and thoughts influence the function and the wiring of the nervous system, and our bodies in turn influence what we sense and feel. To truly understand this, I had to free my own brain from the science I had been taught all these years.

This was not as hard as one might think. I needed better answers. My patients brought symptoms and disorders to me that I could not explain with the anatomy and physiology I knew. They forced me to think differently, outside the conventional realm of traditional medicine, because this type of medicine could not account for the phenomena I was observing day after day.

For example, how could I forget Lyla? I met her years ago, when my team and I were doing research on patients with syringomyelia (a disorder of the nervous system in which cavities, called syrinxes, form within the spinal cord). These patients have damage in large segments of the spinal cord and end up with all kinds of abnormalities (weakness, abnormal reflexes, wobbly gait, bladder problems, pain and loss of sensation from several body regions). Lyla was 38 when I saw her. Since she was 2, her parents would do everything they could to deter her from chewing her fingertips, to no avail. By the time she came to me, she had no fingernails and actually no finger "beds," as she had chewed away the outer part of her fingers. As she was growing up, she had developed clumsiness in her hands and later on her gait became unsteady and she had trouble holding her bladder. At some point, she burned herself badly on her shoulders with a curling iron because she could not feel it. All these symptoms led us to investigations in which the doctors discovered a syrinx throughout the length of Lyla's spinal cord (from the bottom of her skull all the way down to her lower spine). Nobody knew how this syrinx came about. Nevertheless, the neurosurgeons went into her brain and spinal cord and put in a little tube called a shunt to drain the syrinx. This surgery seemed to have stopped the progression of weakness and bladder and bowel problems. But Lyla went on to develop pains in her back and chest, which came and went in spells.

By the time she was admitted to my in-patient unit, there was no syrinx at all to be seen, as it had been drained by the surgeons many years before. But Lyla's spinal cord had become extremely wasted and thin and looked like a tiny rope. If we're talking about anatomical damage, Lyla certainly had it. She had no feeling at all from the neck down. I thought I knew why. With so much spinal cord damage, part of Lyla's pain pathways were destroyed, so she lost her feeling all the way to her feet.

But I was wrong, as my magic drug, amytal, proved. During the administration of the drug, I tested her skin with my pinwheel. Lyla, who to this point had never felt the prick of a needle in her skin, complained bitterly of pain in her hands, feet and part of her abdomen. I was dumbfounded. Here was this woman who suffered unquestionable major damage since birth, who had been chewing senseless her fingers since she was a baby, and now, for a few minutes she could feel pain and actually feel it intensely in body parts that had been insensitive all her life. It just did not make sense. Thank goodness the test was performed in the presence of several team members and Lyla was videotaped. Otherwise, even I might have thought I was imagining things.

Later, the same thing happened again—another patient with a large syrinx and dense anaesthesia in the upper quarter of his body turned nearly normal under amytal. I became then convinced that the lack of sensation my patients with syringomyelia suffered from was not necessarily totally fixed. The evidence was unquestionable: these patients had two kinds of sensory deficits, some of which were permanent (structural or anatomic) and some of which were non-fixed ("dynamic" or functional), superimposed on top of structural damage of the nervous tissue. We then went ahead and published our unbelievable observations.[5]

I was coming slowly to a new understanding of how such sensory deficits could be seen in the context of pain in different patients and under many circumstances: in people with certain types of personalities and certain ways of coping, those under severe stress or who have been confronted by events perceived as life-threatening, in people of certain cultures that are more expressive and intense when it comes to displays of pain and in patients with real anatomical damage. Maybe, I was thinking, the nervous system uses specific blocking mechanisms more often than we think, against external or internal stimuli that are unpleasant, unwanted or frightening. And maybe, as Dr. Nicholson suggested, the way we are brought up affects and influences the kind of wiring we develop and what kinds of mechanisms the nervous system mobilizes to fend off pain or battle stress. Maybe one of these mechanisms is to try to make the painful body parts become insensitive to pain.

Misbehaving Brains

As a result of these investigations into unusual cases, my reputation as someone willing to look into the most bizarre, difficult and incomprehensible situations began to grow. This led to more strange patients finding their way to my clinic.

In late 1999, Monica, 61, was referred to me with a chronic problem with her right shoulder. When she developed pneumonia, the shoulder pain flared up severely, perhaps because of the way she was lying in bed. Within 24 hours, her whole right side went completely numb and weak. Her doctors admitted her to a local hospital, thinking she had had a stroke. Strangely, by the second day in the hospital, her strength and sensation came back, except in her right forearm and hand, which remained completely paralyzed. Her pain, however, had always been confined to her right shoulder. As the paralysis and numbness subsided from the right side, she felt some strange and short-lived pain in the left leg. Then, of all things, her *left* leg became completely numb and paralyzed from the groin. CAT scans of her head did not show any signs of stroke that could explain these bizarre phenomena.

Her doctors were more than puzzled. Monica overheard them talking to her daughter and suggesting that it was all in her head. Furious, she asked for a cab and, against their advice, had herself discharged home in her wheelchair. When she got home, she then boiled water and poured it over her left thigh in a mad effort to "wake up the leg." Within a minute or so, she felt ripples of bizarre sensations in her thigh and the feeling returned, all the way from the top of her thigh to her knee! Below the knee level, however, her left leg remained completely paralyzed and insensitive to touch. Thirteen months later, she showed up at my clinic in her wheelchair.

When I examined Monica, she complained of unbearable right shoulder pain and some burning pain in her left groin. Both her right hand and left leg were cold, terribly swollen, completely insensitive to touch, prick or pinch, and totally paralyzed. A significant point to remember: her groin pain had appeared at the same time as the sensation returned to her thigh when she spilled the boiling water down her leg. A large, discoloured scar across her thigh showed up as testimony to the unusual, drastic method she used to wake up her nervous system.

On videotape, under the administration of sodium amytal, Monica described how she poured boiling water over her thigh and how the sensation came back. With the drug, her ongoing right shoulder and left groin pain disappeared completely, but her shoulder still hurt if I moved it (something that made me suspect a local problem with the joint). As far as sensation was concerned, under amytal, Monica got back all the feeling in her right hand and her ability to move it returned, but not completely, while nothing changed in her left leg. The return of sensation and movement to her hand lasted for a few minutes. Later on, X-rays confirmed arthritis in her shoulder. There was definitely a source of nociceptive pain there, but under no circumstances could it account for the bizarre symptoms Monica had. Thousands of patients suffer from arthritis, but reacting to it with complete loss of sensory and motor function is unheard of. What on earth could explain Monica's reaction to her shoulder pain?

Looking at older records, we realized that something significant had happened to Monica about 10 years before the events that brought her to me. When she was attending her father's funeral back home in Jamaica, it appeared that she suffered what the medical records called a stroke. Her whole left side became paralyzed. After a while she was flown back to Canada and spent a whole year going to physiotherapy. Her side completely recovered from the paralysis and Monica returned to full-time work. We never saw old records confirming the stroke, and since CAT scans and MRIs of her brain taken while she was in my unit had failed to show remnants of old brain damage, I wondered if Monica ever actually had a stroke. So I asked her to describe to me the circumstances of this old "stroke." She explained that she had been very close to her father and had discussed with him being a pallbearer when he died. On the day of the funeral she asked to bear the coffin and was given a middle position, carrying it with her right arm. The coffin was very heavy, so she raised her eyes to the sky and asked: "Father, this is too heavy. Do you want to kill me?" The coffin miraculously became "light as a feather," as she put it. The same night her left side (which did not carry the coffin) became heavier and heavier and next morning it was all dead and paralyzed. Monica, her daughter and I now think that what was called "stroke" at the time was nothing but a bizarre brain behaviour, a game her brain played under conditions of emotional stress during her dad's funeral.

Few of my patients are as extreme as Monica. Most will be like Daniel, Francesca or Fernando. Fernando was born in Chile and moved to Western Canada several years ago. While working at a construction site, he fell off a scaffold from a substantial height (here goes the original frightening event again) and smashed his left elbow. The doctors fixed the broken joint, but Fernando was left with a burning and shooting pain at the site of his forearm all the way down to the last two fingers of his left hand. He had simply damaged the ulnar nerve (the nerve found close to the "funny bone"). He ended up with not one but seven nerve surgeries, with the doctors "cleaning" the nerve from adjacent scar tissue, moving it around and so on, to try to lessen Fernando's pain. Unfortunately, not only did the pain not go away, but during the four years before Fernando came to us, he had gradually lost all movements in his left arm.

When he saw me, Fernando was holding his arm and resting it against his chest. He could not open or clench his fist, extend his elbow or bring his hand to his mouth. He had retrained himself to work with one hand and in the meantime had improved his English and was working part-time as an accountant. He was a flamboyant, loud, olive-skinned man with an explosive speaking manner. Fernando would laugh heartily at the same time as he was complaining bitterly of pain. His deep tendon reflexes were all present and the "bulk" of his muscles was quite good (two things that are incompatible with true paralysis from real neurological damage). Not surprisingly, Fernando had a dense loss of sensation across his whole arm, shoulder, chest and upper back, as well as on his face, but only on the left side. We checked his somatosensory evoked potentials (a test that confirms the integrity of the nervous system from the fingers to the brain) and they were normal. We also ran some electromyographic and nerve conduction studies, which showed only minor abnormality at the ulnar nerve by the elbow. So there was no explanation for the loss of voluntary hand movements and sensation . . . or was there?

I asked Fernando to move his arm. He fixed his eyes intensely on his hand, concentrated, and with great effort he wiggled his fingers maybe a flicker. "My fingers do not want to move," he said. "My brain orders them to go, but it seems as if they do not want or do not know how to obey." What he was telling me was not unheard of. In many cases, patients would complain bitterly that the insensitive but painful body part did not seem capable of moving spontaneously. In such cases, it is as if the patient had lost the know-how to execute a movement even when imagining the action in his or her brain.

Under sodium amytal, Fernando's pain diminished dramatically within minutes, while at the same time sensation started coming back. By the end of the session, his pain was almost all gone and sensation had completely returned, but he still had trouble initiating movements in the motionless arm and hand.

So I supported his arm with my own hands and while he was looking, I moved his fingers gently toward his mouth. I coaxed and encouraged him: "You can do it, come on, try and I'll help." He looked at his fingers and concentrated hard. I moved his hand from the chest to the mouth again, and again, and again. With each movement Fernando's own muscles kicked in and contributed more. After a few tries I let him do it on his own, while I congratulated him and assured him that as he was moving his arm repeatedly, his brain was switching to "normal." To his amazement, he was able to move his arm and feel the skin of his face and his limb, something he had not been able to do for four years. But by the time he left my unit three days later, the anaesthesia had returned and his movements were all lost. Nevertheless, his pain was not nearly as bad.

I set Fernando up with a physiotherapist and explained what was happening to Fernando's brain. Fernando started coming regularly to the outpatient physiotherapy clinic and became fond of his therapist, grateful for her skills and guidance. He worked hard at the gym and at home, convinced he could "retrain his brain." Week after week Fernando regained more and more movement. First he got back his shoulder movements, some weeks later his elbow, and finally, after about six months, his hand came back to life. Up to the time his hand motion returned, his anaesthesia was dense and impenetrable. But when the hand movements came back, Fernando (to both his and my surprise) started feeling his whole arm and hand again, except for a strip along the inside part of his forearm and his last two fingers. In other words, when the anaesthesia that blanketed the left side of his face, his left shoulder, arm and hand was lifted, it left behind what was there in the first place—a strip of lost sensation exactly in the territory of the injured nerve. Medicines that had never helped before were now effective. Small doses of a tricyclic antidepressant provided Fernando with considerable pain relief.

As I tried to understand what had happened in Fernando's body, I followed a path that in retrospect seems straightforward but that at the time was something of a revelation for me. Fernando had suffered a physical injury in the past, which in turn provoked his brain to react in a bizarre way to try to combat the pain. As the brain's peculiar reaction slowly lifted, Fernando's true injury began to reveal itself. Dealing with the original nerve injury then became easier than dealing with a bizarre and unpredictable brain.

Fernando finally left to return to Western Canada. Before he left, he sent a letter to the vice president of the hospital: "The accomplishments have been remarkable. I now can raise my arm. . . . I can bend my elbow and I can even grab small things with my fingers. I never imagined I could move my arm again. Now I am regaining my confidence and maybe I can restart my own business, the same way it was before I had this accident." I was exhilarated. My job is quite hard and often unrewarding, as I deal with everybody's complex pain problems, and I cannot brag that I often manage to turn the tables. Stories with a happy ending like Fernando's are the fuel that keeps me going.

But what exactly is happening to the brain and the nervous system of patients like Fernando? The questions that beg for answers are endless. What mobilizes these types of sensory and motor phenomena? Is it fear? Duress? Pain itself? Is the makeup of our own personality or the way we cope responsible for these phenomena? Are they created by intractable pain or is it that the pain becomes intractable once they show up—or both? Why can I reverse them with amytal? What is so special about this drug and what does it do to the brain? Why did Daniel and Fernando respond consistently by shedding their anaesthesia under amytal, while with Monica things improved only in her hand for a few minutes? Does this mean that in some people these "dynamic" deficits become permanent and fixed after some time?

I became convinced that the answers to these questions were all locked up in the brain. When (at last) we got our newer fMRI magnet, Dr. Karen Davis started studying my patients in a systematic way. Daniel was tested again. The data we obtained from his brain were the same as what we had gotten four years before. By now, our findings could not be viewed as "technical artifacts" with the fMRI machine; we simply had to accept that Daniel's right cortex was either non-responsive or would become deactivated (in other words, the brain activity was less than normal) after stimulation of the anaesthetic leg. (See the drawings on page 190.) Monica's findings were the same as those of three other patients. In all the cases we studied, the primary somatosensory cortex was either not activated at all or deactivated when we tested the anaesthetic and painful limb. In addition, there were other odd changes in many other brain areas (thalamus, posterior parietal cortex, prefrontal cortex and anterior cingulate gyrus).[6] There was no question whatsoever that we had confirmation of

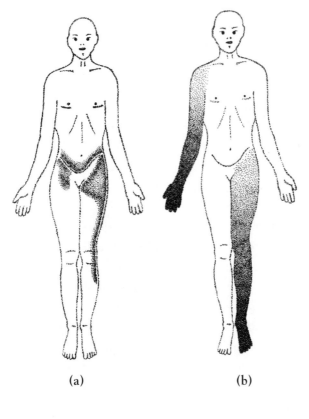

The shaded areas in these body maps correspond to Daniel's pain and loss of sensation. In (a), the shaded area represents Daniel's pains, which are much worse in his left leg. In (b), the artist has marked the regions of sensory loss. Darker shades correspond to intense loss of all skin feeling. Notice that Daniel's right arm cannot "feel" and he has no pain at all.

(a)   (b)

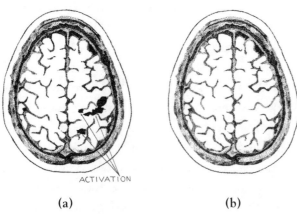

ACTIVATION

(a)   (b)

Artistic rendering of the fMRI views of Daniel's brain. In (a), Daniel's brain is properly activated when his normal right leg is stimulated. In (b), Daniel's brain remains inactive when the anaesthetic left leg is tested.

what I had been saying for so many years about my patients who had "lost" all sensation in the affected parts of their bodies. Something was blocking their sensation, and that something was happening in their brains.

Treating Dysfunctional Brains

Daniel was the first patient to make me think "brain dysfunction," and the one who taught me the most. He actually did have a physical cause for some pain in his left leg, the scarring across the left fifth lumbar root—in medical terms, nerve root fibrosis. But this wasn't enough to explain the massive loss of sensation. So I came up with a novel hypothesis in an effort to explain what seemed to be unexplainable. In my way of thinking, the pain experienced by patients like Daniel, Fernando and Monica had initiated a cascade of reactions:

1. The pain makes the brain mobilize some form of "pain blocking" circuits or inhibition, in an attempt to "shut down" the pain. This inhibition of pain is supposed to be achieved by turning off sensation and often movement.
2. The process, however, fails. While it shuts down sensation (and often movement as in the case of Fernando and Monica), the pain escapes and actually becomes worse and debilitating. In other words, the brain experiences reorganizational changes that we call *plasticity*, but because these changes are not useful, I call it "bad" or "maladaptive" plasticity.
3. In some patients these plastic changes in the brain are temporary and the inhibition is reversed with amytal or with treatments like the one Fernando received; in others the changes soon become fixed and permanent.
4. Often, the magnitude of the original physical injuries may be quite small, but once the cascade of reactions is initiated, they take on a life of its own.

The hundreds of patients I have seen with these deficits of varying degree and severity have convinced me that I am right: It is only in certain individuals that the brain tries to get rid of pain by switching off sensation (and at times movement). Usually the sensory deficit and the motor weakness target the pain in the *affected* side. But whatever bizarre process the brain evokes, it does not do a good job. Not only does this process fail to remove the pain, but once it appears, the pain becomes more severe, as happened with Francesca, Daniel and Fernando. Even worse, this process may hit targets *at random,* producing paralysis and anaesthesia in another limb and not the one with the problem, as in Monica's case.

The concept of "maladaptive neuroplasticity"—an inhibitory, top-down process generated by my patients' brains—is an attempt to block their pain. While the process worked from the top down, their pain most often was generated from the bottom up, for example by an injury, which could be minuscule and insignificant, such as a muscle sprain. In my mind and that of team psychologist Dr. Nicholson, two things were of paramount importance in the appearance of: the conditions around the time of the injury and the way the individual had learned to cope with stress. Maybe these two factors somehow dictate whether these inhibitory processes would set in and what they would do. This was a revolutionary hypothesis. Our research was leading us to think there is a much more direct and powerful relationship between the mind and the body— the concept that our feelings and the ways we cope and view the world, and for that matter our upbringing and our culture, affect the connections within our nervous system. The idea that one's brain can tell a part of the body to ache miserably—or for that matter to feel nothing at all—has been around for centuries, but we were now taking a long and hard look at thinking brains by using the most modern imaging techniques.

But as I began turning these ideas over in my mind, I had patients who needed treatment. I could not afford to wait for years of research to tell me what to do. I felt I had to manage their pain based on our hypothesis, and to experiment with "aberrant and misbehaving" brains. For Fernando, a combination of goal-oriented physical treatments, the support and encouragement he received by a devoted and understanding therapist, and his conviction after what we taught him that his problem truly could be fixed had worked. But what about Daniel? What could work for him?

I had another daring thought: In Daniel's case, maybe targeting the nerve root fibrosis with a spinal stimulator could sufficiently block the painful impulses from the leg to the brain, and finally advise the brain that this business of inhibition was not needed anymore. So I approached the interventional team in my hospital—a team of anaesthetists and neurosurgeons—and asked them to give Daniel a trial of spinal stimulation. The Workers' Compensation Board in Ontario (now called the Workplace Safety and Insurance Board) approved my request and funding was in place. After a long time on a waiting list, Daniel finally got his trial.

For a successful trial, spinal stimulation should generate tingling throughout the painful limb. The surgeons thread electrodes on the surface of the spinal cord through a needle at the back of the spine. Then they attach them to an external device and leave them in for a few days, to see if the pain can be blocked. If during the trial the patient experiences substantial pain relief, then the stimulator is implanted permanently under the skin. Daniel was given a week for the trial.

Unfortunately, nothing happened during the first few days. Daniel felt a tingling down his left leg, but the pain was still there. Daniel, a highly anxious man, would phone me from home nearly every day to update me. Then, one Monday morning, a few days after the start of the trial, and a day before he was to see the interventional team, he called me again to confess what he had done the night before. In his despair for the lack of response, he opened up the device and tampered with the wires. All of a sudden, he experienced at least 70 to 80 per cent pain relief! With this kind of result, when he saw the surgeons two days later, they had no other option but to implant the stimulator. Was this abrupt pain relief a placebo effect that reflected Daniel's desire to make it work? The answer in my mind was a resounding yes, but Daniel wanted the stimulator so much that I had no intention of even communicating my doubts to the surgeons, or to him for that matter. He got the device implanted in his back early in May 2001.

Bingo! The pain was reduced dramatically, as he kept the stimulator working almost constantly. Daniel threw out all his painkillers, put his cane out of sight and started living. He would strut into my office, slim, swift, elegant and excited, almost unable to put into words how it felt to be able to ride a bicycle and swim with his young son. Daniel also rediscovered his sexuality and would overflow with joy describing how he was trying to "make up for lost years." This was wonderful in terms of treating his pain, but terrible for my hypothesis, which seemed to have been thrown out the window. Blocking pain impulses from the spinal cord to the brain did not change the complete loss of sensation in his leg, which I had attributed to "maladaptive neuroplasticity."

But by late July, about three months after the implantation of the spinal stimulator, Daniel announced to me that he started having bizarre flashes of pins and needles in his left foot, the foot he had not felt for eight years. And, by August, the unbelievable occurred: Daniel got back sensation when he was touched, pricked with a pin and pinched, all the way down to his foot, with the exception of a strip of numbness at the territory of the scarred root. He was overjoyed and so was I. In my heart, I felt that the pain relief and the return of sensation were more the results of Daniel's desire to get better than the effect of the stimulator on his brain.

A job came up with the public transit system. It needed bus drivers. Daniel, through his years of hardship, had returned to school and obtained a diploma as information systems programmer with honours (a copy of this is prominently displayed on the walls of my office, a gift from Daniel). He applied for the driver's job, planning to do it for one year and then perhaps advance to the system's central computer offices. Daniel was called for an interview. He became obsessed with getting the job. He wanted so badly to get back into the workforce that this desire dominated every waking hour of his day. I supported him with all my heart, crossing my fingers and hoping for the best because he had suffered so much. But it was not that easy.

By mid-September, Daniel started complaining of a new pain in his left buttock and hip after he slipped and fell on the floor. The pain mounted and Daniel returned to opioids. The leg sensation, however, was still there. Finally, a CAT scan with myelogram was done, only to show that the electrode tip of the spinal stimulator had moved after the fall and was touching his left first lumbar root, the root that exactly innervates the buttock area. Daniel came to see me in both physical and emotional agony: "I must pass my medical test, do something to help me." The company knew that Daniel had "failed back syndrome" and an implanted stimulator, but did not care as long as he could do all the things a driver is supposed to do. So I gave him a couple of injections of opioids to carry him through. At the medical, Daniel bit his lip, held his breath, smiled and passed. He would have to wait a few months for his turn to undergo training. Shortly after, Daniel showed up at the hospital's emergency department with excruciating hip pain and was admitted to neurosurgery. Next day, he was taken to the operating room, and his precious stimulator was removed. I coached him before the surgery: "Don't despair. Maybe the brief trial of implanted stimulation was enough to reverse this inhibition. Maybe everything will continue to be fine after the device is gone."

As a matter of fact, everything did turn out to be fine. The hip pain disappeared, and the nearly painless leg with all its normal feeling, was still there. But the curse that had haunted Daniel for the past eight years did not want to let go. He developed a serious wound infection in his back. Pus was dripping from the incision, to the point that the doctors left the wound open to drain, put him on IV antibiotics and sent him home with daily nursing care. But his leg was still holding, against all odds. Finally, Daniel got his work training and got the job. But once he started working, the sensation from the left foot was gradually lost. Daniel was putting himself through tremendous demands with long hours of sitting, refusing to take any painkillers. I was thinking about him and was worried: he had a screwed-up back with nerve root scarring and a "funny" brain that in my estimation could go "berserk" any time again. I viewed his brain as a time bomb packed with pain messages, ready to explode under stress or threats to Daniel's bodily and mental integrity.

Against my predictions, six months after the removal of the stimulator, and three months into the job, despite indescribable physical hardship and profound stress, Daniel held on, counting the months until he could make it to the central office. He was a fighter, for whom succeeding at work was the greatest desire. For a while I thought that I was too pessimistic.

Then something awful happened. While driving the bus, Daniel was assaulted twice in three weeks, on the same night route, by drunks and potheads. Understandably, he became frightened. He developed signs and symptoms of post-traumatic stress reaction and was afraid to drive the night route on which the assaults had taken place. When he came to see me for follow-up, he knew it was his brain that was letting him down. Within these few weeks, he had lost all forms of sensation from the knee to the foot. "But I am still good, doctor," he said looking at me with big eyes, hoping I would support his statement. "I still have the sensation in my thigh and buttock, so not everything is lost, right?" I asked him what he really wanted, as his employer had just given him the week off. He wanted his job back and asked me to clear him to return to work. I consented, but with a warning: he should not be placed back on the night route, not at least for a while. I had to protect him from any further emotional troubles of this sort.

He returned back to work a week later, driving his bus. But I am sure I have not heard the last of Daniel. He and I have a history of sorts. If and when the anaesthesia shrinks again (perhaps when Daniel makes it to his computer position), I will be able to test his brain with fMRI again. I know I have helped him a lot as a doctor, but so far, he has taught me a lot as a patient. I have learned from him about how we can change the behaviour of such bizarre brains, and that it is "bad stress" (like the assaults) and not "good stress" (like physical fatigue from his work, the work he considers a ticket to his target) that sets up these short circuits.

Beyond Pain, Beyond Traditional Medicine

Blair was 37 when he was sent to me by a specialist who was confused by this man's problem. Blair had suffered a peroneal nerve injury (damage to the nerve running from the outside of his knee to his foot) during surgery to repair a cartilage in his left knee torn 20 years before. This type of nerve injury left Blair unable to bend his foot upward. He ended up wearing a special brace to help him lift the foot off the ground during walking, and he had surgery to tie together some tendons on the top of the foot. Blair had gone on like this for 18 years before he saw me with a half-paralyzed foot. As the brace and the surgery helped him walk, he went on with his life, working for the local telephone company. Surprisingly, from the time of the surgery Blair's leg had become extremely numb and insensitive from just above the knee all the way to the foot. He could not sense the floor, but he really did not care. He got used to this dense and painless numbness, and none of his physicians questioned why he had lost all the sensation from the leg, and not just the part innervated by the injured nerve.

But two years before Blair's referral to me, he slipped and twisted his knee again. He felt acute, shearing pain and his knee swelled up. Although he went for physiotherapy and took Aspirin-like medications, the knee pain did not seem to improve; it actually got worse. Yet the anaesthesia and paralysis of the leg gradually diminished. By six weeks after the new knee injury they were completely gone.

The doctor who referred him to me tested him with new electrophysiological studies. He documented old remnants of the nerve injury. But if nerves are to recover, they do so within a year or two. How come Blair got back the sensation and the movement 18 whole years after the original nerve damage? Did it really take that many years for Blair's nerve to heal? It just did not make sense.

On examination, Blair walked with a slight limp because his left knee was hurting. But there were no signs of paralysis. He had a cold, purple knee very sensitive to touch, with a strip of reduced sensation in the outside of the leg, exactly what one would have expected from a peroneal nerve damage. Blair's picture now was a textbook case of "causalgia."

"Doctor," he pleaded, "can you please take away all this pain and give me back what I had for so many years? I did not mind a dead and weak leg, but I mind very much this unbearable pain.

"By the way," he continued, "do you know what is happening to me now?"
I thought I knew.

"I am afraid, Blair, that you have now what you were supposed to experience 20 years ago, when you had the nerve damage. You were protected then by a bizarre game played by your brain. It blocked the pain by exchanging it for a senseless and half-paralyzed leg. But when you twisted your knee again, the new acute pain jolted your brain and woke it up!"

I treated Blair's pain with appropriate neuropathic medications and strong painkillers. The effect was only partial. Today, he is permanently off work and on disability. As he told me, if he ever had a choice, he would bring back the anaesthesia and paralysis to get rid of his pain.

These types of sensory abnormalities and paralysis are hallmarks of what doctors for hundreds of years have called "hysterical" symptoms. *Hysteria* is a term that originated from the Greek word *hystero* or womb. It was coined by Hippocrates, the great Greek doctor of antiquity, the father of modern medicine. In the beginning, hysteria was considered somehow a women's condition, generated "by the motion of the uterus in the body." This condition included paralysis, muscle contractures, anaesthesia and other unusual symptoms. But our understanding of hysteria advanced in the late nineteenth century thanks to Jean-Martin Charcot, the great French neurologist, and his students, one of whom was the famous Sigmund Freud. Charcot considered "hysterical" hemiplegia (paralysis of one side of the body) or anaesthesia examples of *physiological dysfunction* in certain brain areas, and called them "dynamic aberrations" of brain function. These phenomena did not have an anatomical or structural basis, as autopsies of such patients failed to show damage in the corresponding brain areas. Charcot, who was the first one to describe "hysterical phenomena" in men too, felt that psychological factors were important in generating all these strange brain behaviours. Freud also discussed them extensively and observed that "hysteria behaves as though neuroanatomy does not exist." In other words, by the nineteenth century hysteria was viewed as a neurological disorder, and psychological factors were recognized as seeming to play an important role as well.

It is my feeling that my patients and thousands of others around the world with such strange anaesthetic responses and paralysis are rewriting our books of physiology, moving beyond pain and beyond conventional medical knowledge and understanding. When the late Dr. Patrick Wall heard me speaking about these bizarre brain games in one of my talks a few years ago, he told me I should read a book called *A Leg to Stand On* by Dr. Oliver Sacks, the well-known neurologist and author of several best sellers.[7] Sacks described a very frightening experience that occurred when he was hiking alone in Norway in the 1970s. He was chased by a bull and he ran in "mad panic," as he put it, for his life. He fell and severed his left quadriceps, the strong muscle that supports the knee. At the same time he shattered the nerve to this muscle. The event was terribly frightening, as the doctor faced a true life-or-death situation. A couple of days later, he was flown to England, his severed muscle was reattached and his whole leg was put in a cast from the groin almost to the foot.

For the first two days, Sacks experienced excruciating pain and needed morphine. Rather suddenly, on the third day, the pain disappeared. As it subsided, Sacks realized in horror that he had "forgotten" how to make the leg move, or that he even owned a leg, as the limb had become completely paralyzed from the groin to the ankle, sparing the foot. Two weeks later, when the cast was removed, Sacks was bewildered even more. He found out that his whole leg—every inch that had been in the cast—was literally "dead." The leg "felt like wax." As he describes in his book, "I squeezed it, pinched it and pulled a hair." Horrified, he realized that he had no sensation whatsoever. This could not be explained by the injury to the nerve of the quadriceps muscle.

Ultimately, after several weeks of convalescence, Sacks conquered both the anaesthesia and the paralysis of his leg and went on to near-complete recovery. Five years later, however, he sustained a similar injury to his other leg when he slipped at a gas station. But this event was not life-threatening and this time, he did not experience anaesthesia or paralysis.

I think that the immense fear Dr. Sacks felt when the Norway accident occurred, together with the acute pain of injury, set up changes in his brain, changes that are very similar to what my patients display. Putting it all together, the brain is strange and sometimes unpredictable. Most times it behaves the way the books say it should. But other times, it works in incomprehensible ways to shut off pain and all kinds of other frightening and unpleasant stimuli, physical or emotional. I am convinced that at times of intense emotions, the brain in some individuals can shut off sensation and movement, vision and hearing and the ability to talk or even to remember.

A few years ago, I was describing patients like Daniel and Fernando to a group of hard-core experimental neuroscientists who study animals that suffer from nerve damage to their legs. Their work is very different from mine, given the fact I study humans, who are awake and have more complex brains. Usually, scientists stare at me with blank eyes when I talk to them about "maladaptive neuroplasticity" and misbehaving brains that can shut down sensation, movement, vision and hearing. But that night, I found a great ally to support such a concept, as one of the scientists told us his own story.

When this scientist was young, his father told him how he had witnessed a fatal factory fire. Because of what he saw, his father taught my friend to always find out where the fire exit was located in any structure, be it in an office, a theatre or in an airplane. My colleague learned not only to locate fire exits wherever he went, but also to sit on aisles in a theatre, close to a fire exit. Once, as bad luck would have it, the theatre where he was attending a performance caught fire. He told me about his own feeling—mad fear—and how he went nearly blind in an instant. Actually, he lost all his visual fields except a narrow tunnel of sight in the middle, which he used to scan his environment to find the fire exit. When he managed to get out of the theatre, his vision returned.

"What you tell me makes sense," he said. "In my panic my occipital cortex [the part of brain that controls vision] was partially blocked, and it left me with a narrow tube of vision, enough to concentrate on finding the exit." He knew he did not imagine this, but he had never fully understood what had happened. Now he was able to connect his experience to the concept.

In my way of thinking, when it comes to pain, the magnitude of the original injury does not seem to dictate the degree of sensory and motor inhibition. I believe strongly that it is more the *circumstances* under which an injury occurs and the way we handle emotions or cope with everyday life (in other words the *fabric of our personalities and our coping mechanisms* when we face stress) that matter more in the generation of the bizarre sensory and motor phenomena I have described. Beyond our genes and our physical makeup or the magnitude of a physical trauma, our emotions, our culture and our personality influence profoundly our neural circuits and the body's reactions. In some of my patients, like Francesca, although the injury is insignificant, emotions fly high, the expressions of pain are intense and the disability profound. These patients would traditionally fit the conventional description of hysteria, and multidisciplinary cognitive-behavioural treatment approaches may be more beneficial to them than injections, drugs or surgery alone.

In other patients, however, the injury is substantial and needs to be addressed first, in the hope that the brain subsequently will be convinced to "lift" the inhibition. In most, the reality is somewhere in between and the management of pain must at all times address the physical, psychological and emotional components of pain and disability.

We are only scratching the surface right now. As we unravel the mysteries of the thinking and feeling brain, we will have to use tools such as imaging studies to redraw our neurological maps. We will have to rethink connections and circuits.

And we will have to teach our medical students that everything is possible when body and mind interact.

Eleven

THE GOOD, THE BAD
AND THE UGLY

People often wonder whether doctors work harder to treat patients they like compared with patients they don't like. While I can't speak for all doctors, I know that I try hard to help everyone who comes to me with pain. But on several occasions, I have found that the interactions with some patients can take their toll.

The Violent Patient

In the 1980s, at the start of my career, I had an office in the basement of a medical building across the street from the Toronto Western Hospital. My office and the even tinier examining room faced an open rectangular space housing a physiotherapy department. My assistant Anna occupied another little room at the entrance to the physiotherapy department. All patients would have to sit down with her for a few minutes so she could collect appropriate information (name, address, health card number and so on) and then she would bring the patient and the file to me. Once, I was fiddling with some files and waiting for the first patient of the day, when Anna ran hysterically toward my office: "Dr. Mailis, can you speak to this guy? I was trying to ask him information about his father, your patient, when he told me to shove the papers in my ass!"

Alarmed, I stood up. Behind Anna, a monster emerged. He was in his late 30s or early 40s, at least 1.9 metres (6 feet, 5 inches) tall. Within a flash I estimated that he was probably 136 kilograms (300 pounds). His head was shaved, he had a long, black beard, his belly stuck out and he was wearing a muscle shirt that revealed some humungous biceps decorated with long, intricate tattoos. Over his shirt he wore a studded leather vest; to complete the picture he sported leather pants and heavy boots with chains at the back of the heels. He immediately reminded me of scary movies and biker gangs.

"What is going on?" I asked.

The monster replied angrily: "This crazy woman wants all this information. Can't she find it in the papers?"

"No, sir, this information must be given to us by the patient or his guardian. We are not going to search the files for it. And besides, your manners are unacceptable. You are not allowed to behave like this."

"Listen, woman," the big guy counterattacked, "I am a biker and I can behave like a pig anywhere I want!"

I lost it. I took a few steps in front of my old oak desk, pointed my finger at him and stamped the floor, yelling at the top of my lungs: "You might be a pig, but this is not a pigsty. Get out of here. Get out of here unless you apologize."

"I am not apologizing to anyone. You are a bunch of crazies," he snapped back. I walked aggressively toward him, blinded by anger, and then the monster stepped back, and back . . . and back. He turned around and literally grabbed an old man by the shoulder, who, it was clear, was his poor father whom I was supposed to see.

"Let's get out of here, they are all mad," the big son shouted, and he pulled his father behind him, like a sack of potatoes.

The old man mumbled, "I really don't understand why they kick me out of every doctor's office."

"Sir," I said with pity, "it is not you. I will be glad to see you if you come without him."

They left. Dazed, I sat down, trying to control my anger. Stephen, a young physiotherapist who had witnessed the whole event, came to talk to me.

"Didn't you realize he could have hurt you?" he said. "One blow would have thrown you over your desk. I was so scared."

During those tense moments it hadn't occurred to me that the big ugly man could have attacked me physically—I was far too blind with rage to think or reason. But my rage had obviously worked. The sight of me pounding the floor with my heels, pointing a finger and walking toward him while yelling must have taken the man by surprise.

I placed an urgent call to the family physician who had referred the old man, located somewhere in Northern Ontario. He was deeply apologetic: "It's the same old story. This man has twin sons and you saw one of them. They are both members of a criminal motorcycle gang and they terrorize our community. I am so sorry you got the full force of his wrath. I don't know where else to send the old man anymore; the brothers create the same troubles everywhere."

This was one of my early contacts with violence in my field of work. The biker's picture haunted me for a while. Many years later, when I got my own Harley-Davidson motorcycle and began riding, it became clear to me that the wonderful men and women I meet and ride with have no relationship to this big fool or, I suppose, his twin brother.

During the 20 years of my career, I have had a few more brushes with violence. Michael had been sent to me in the early 1990s by his family doctor. He had suffered some serious injuries, including a head injury, after his snow-mobile crashed into a tree trunk. He had been unconscious for several days and was left with some neuropathic pain in his arm. But in my opinion, his most significant problem was his personality change after the head injury.

Michael had no control over his anger and frustration, and his memory was quite impaired. Nevertheless, he did not come back to see me for at least four years. Then out of the blue, he asked to see me again. I knew something was wrong with him the moment he entered my room.

"Well, Michael, what has been going on with you for so many years?" I asked.

His voice rose fast, the speed of his speech intensified and he became sweaty and flushed: "It's all your doing. You and the other doctors are all incompetent. You left me with this pain and you do not care."

I had no idea what he was talking about, as I had seen him only once and had sent all my recommendations to his family doctor, to be carried out where he lived, hours away from Toronto. I tried to calm him, but to no avail. He started pacing the office, talking louder and louder. I was getting quite uncomfortable, as in those years I did not have any martial arts skills with which to protect myself. Anna, from across the corridor, must have heard the yelling and she phoned me.

"Everything all right?" she asked.

"No, I don't think so," I replied. She sensed the anxiety in my voice and said, "Don't worry, I'll get security."

The waiting felt endless. When the two security guards finally walked in— a middle-aged man and a younger rather short woman—Michael became bewildered. They tried to calm him, but they too were unsuccessful. Sensing impending danger, the female security guard slipped out of my office to call the police. I have no recollection of the exact sequence or duration of events. I recall only feeling trapped behind my desk. As the other security guard tried to guide me toward the door, Michael, enraged, raised one of the chairs and threw it against the wall. The heavy chair left a deep indentation as it bounced on the wall and then the floor. By then two police officers had arrived. I recall only the yelling as I was sitting in Anna's office, rather shaky, while the police dealt with Michael. Then Michael passed by me, hands shackled, arms held by the police. I never saw him again, but I never forgot him either.

Violence in pain clinics like mine is not that rare. In a talk I attended in the United States in November 2000, a group of researchers reported on chronic pain patients who think of harming others. Such patients with violent thoughts can represent up to 13 per cent of all those attending a chronic pain program.[1] But of course, violent thoughts can be very different from violent acts. Events like the episode with Michael can be counted on the fingers of one hand in my own career span. But while these episodes are rare, verbally abusive and obnoxious patients unfortunately are not.

The ones who usually take the brunt of such abuse are my front-line workers, the secretarial and administrative staff. Anna has been sworn at, told off or even spat on by patients who demand appointments, papers for their claims or narcotics. I have a very strong—and uncompromising—attitude toward protecting my staff, so I often get involved in settling the issues. At times, though, the target of the wrath is me.

The Obnoxious Patient

Eileen was a registered nurse in one of our city's teaching hospitals. Her family doctor was at a loss to explain why she was still out of work because of what sounded like a minor sprain of the shoulder tendons, after an incident with an agitated patient. She was in her late 30s, single, well dressed and emotionally restrained. After she was referred to me and I began taking a detailed history, Eileen suddenly burst into tears that she didn't manage to control for the duration of the interview. I tried to figure out why she was crying. She vehemently denied pain but she would not tell me where this torrent of tears was coming from. At the end of my examination, having found very little, I suggested certain exercises to maintain her range of movements and the use of a TENS machine to subdue the pain. I sent her doctor a note and I suggested that maybe her tears were a sign of depression.

Eileen came for follow-up two months later. She started by telling me how thankful she was. Exercises and TENS had worked miracles and she was to return back to work shortly. And then her facial expression changed. She looked me straight in the eyes and her voice resonated through the room: "You know, I asked my family physician to give me a copy of the note you sent him about me. You had no right whatsoever to say that I was depressed. I asked about you, and some people told me you are arrogant, condescending and rude." I was speechless.

She reached into her bag, pulled out a piece of paper and laid it on my desk. "Take a look," she ordered. The paper was titled "The evolution of the man." There were four pictures of footprints on it. The first one showed the footprints of an ape, the second picture the footprints of bare human feet, the third one those of a man's shoes and the fourth one footprints of a woman's high heels. She pointed to the ape footprints and then to the woman's footprints and continued mercilessly: "When I came here the other time, I saw no difference between the ape and the woman!"

I managed to collect my thoughts and force a smile on my face. "I am glad, at least, that my treatment helped you." Her face lit up with a smile. "It took me time to overcome my fear of you, but I am so glad I was able to tell you how I feel about you. Make sure," she added with an abrupt tone, "you send a note to my physician, the Workers' Compensation and a copy to me as well, so I know what you are saying about me." She slammed the door and left me dazed; I really felt as if I had been whacked with a baseball bat. I walked into Anna's office.

"What in the name of God happened to you? You are so pale," Anna said. For the life of me I had not been able to understand what I had done to provoke such wrath.

"You don't need to try," Anna consoled me. "She is obviously quite disturbed because I cannot see anything to justify her behaviour. But we'll fix her! You just dictate a note for today's follow-up but make sure that you include details of your encounter with her." So I did. I dictated a brief follow-up note indicating that Ms. So-and-so had improved remarkably with the treatment I had recommended and she was returning to work. At the end I added a little postscript. "By the way, Ms. So-and-so indicated to me that she did not like me as a physician and a professional and brought me a copy of four pairs of footprints . . . ." The next paragraph gave the whole story. At the end I attached the page with the footprints and sent a copy to workers' compensation, the referring physician and the patient herself. I never heard from Eileen again. I suppose she was too embarrassed to come after me.

The "Sexy" Patient

François was short, bald, chubby, 40 and single—"not exactly an oil painting," as they say in England. He was referred to me for intermittent disabling leg pains. Two diseases are the primary culprits for leg pains that arise from walking: vascular claudication (ischemia of the legs due to poor blood supply caused by peripheral vascular disease) and neurogenic claudication (pinched nerve roots at the level of the lumbar spine due to a narrow spinal canal). To help François, I had to first take a thorough history, asking questions about pain and associated symptoms. A good pain doctor must ask about all kinds of functions that may be affected by pain and clogged blood vessels or pinched nerves. So with a straight face (I had practised early in my career, as this was a difficult topic for me), I asked François about his ability to have erections, since erectile abnormalities may be caused by poor blood supply, which could also generate his leg pains. François sounded hesitant. "Well, hmmmm, well, no problems there." But then he paused. "To tell you the truth doctor, hmmm, there is a problem there . . . you know . . . not because I can't get it up . . . but because there is no girlfriend, you know." As he seemed to want to talk more about his love life—or lack of it—than his medical condition, I changed the subject rather quickly. "Sir, please follow me to the examining room," I said. "Here is a hospital gown. Please remain with your underwear but use this gown. I'll be back in five minutes."

I proceeded with a thorough examination, studying his gait, the range of movement in his spine, reflexes and muscle strength and so on. As he was lying on the examining bed, there was one more examination I had to complete to rule out vascular claudication and peripheral vascular disease. "Sir," I explained, "I must feel your pulses in the feet, behind your knees and in your groin to make sure you have good circulation." By the time my fingers reached François's groin to feel the pulse, a distinct vertical bulge became very prominent under the hospital gown. François grew sweaty and flushed and all of a sudden the sign "red alert" started ringing in my head.

"Sir," I said, gasping, "we are finished. Please get dressed and come to the office." Rather late.

"You see what you did," François yelled. I ran to Anna's office to catch my breath and gave him time to cool down. The consultation was terminated quickly, and thankfully there was no follow-up.

The Emotionally Disturbed Patient

Neda was a bank manager in her mid-30s. She had a long history of abdominal pain for which she had had her gall bladder removed, plus some additional abdominal surgery, but to no avail. Tests did not show what was wrong. A few sessions of acupuncture did make the pain go away; but the pain returned four months later when she found she was pregnant with her third child. After the delivery Neda's abdominal pains continued to occur in spells, exactly the same way they used to happen before her gall bladder was removed. The spells were so serious that she had to visit the local emergency a few times every month for injections of Demerol. She had been unable to work for two years. At home she was dependent on her husband, who was doing the cooking, shopping, laundry and cleaning the bathroom, while her mother-in-law was looking after the second child and the baby. Her 13-year-old son was assisting his father in house duties as well.

Having all that household help may sound like domestic bliss, but she continued to complain of intractable pain. Her physician referred her to our clinic, and I offered Neda admission to the in-patient unit, as I needed to explore both the physical and psycho-emotional aspects of her pain. She assured me she was taking only a few pills of quick-release morphine per day, as her doctor prescribed. As is customary, she gave her medications to the nurses when she was admitted, to be locked in the nursing station, and would receive only what I formally prescribed, again through the nurse who is assigned to her.

However, when I made rounds at 11 a.m. the next day, Neda did not seem to be able to wake up. She responded with some incomprehensible sounds when her name was called. It was clear she was deeply sedated. Alarmed, I reviewed all the medications we had prescribed for her. None was strong enough to explain her severe sedation. I ordered the nurses to withhold all medications and watch her. About four hours later I got a call from the ward. Would I speak to the head nurse, the ward clerk asked.

"Dr. Mailis," the head nurse said, "You would not believe what happened. Two of the nurses went to help Neda to the bathroom because she was so unstable on her feet. When they got her out of the bed, they found a syringe full of something under her covers, and another one empty."

I told the head nurse to hold onto the syringes and say nothing to Neda. I made urgent arrangements to have the content of the syringes analyzed. Within an hour and a half, I received a fax from the toxicology lab. The filled syringe contained a large dose of Demerol and the empty one had traces of Valium and Demerol. I called an urgent meeting of the team. The psychologist and psychiatrist had already seen Neda. They found her manipulative and emotionally unstable. The family situation was a real mess, as there were lots of conflicts, particularly with the mother-in-law. We all agreed not to confront Neda directly at this stage, but to suggest gradual discontinuation of her morphine and replacement by non-addictive painkillers. We felt she needed antidepressants, intense counselling and psychotherapy. We knew that the only visitor she received every day was her husband. This meant, of course, that he was the only suspect for bringing the syringes.

Unfortunately, things turned ugly. Neda's roommate in the hospital told her that the nurses had found the syringes tangled in Neda's bedsheets. Neda, who was still an in-patient, became enraged. She called the police that same night and threatened suicide if we were not going to take her pain away. We brought the Emergency Psychiatry Service to monitor her. It was obvious that Neda was deeply disturbed and that there were major psychosocial issues at home. She accused the nurses of "conspiring to frame her," and she took out her wrath on me, accusing me of being totally responsible for "my conspiring nurses." Neda made numerous phone calls to the police, the hospital's public relations office and to my secretary, who passed her on to me several times. No matter how hard I tried to mellow her, she would jump from being kind and gentle to wildly angry within seconds. Her husband called several times too. My whole day was literally shot to hell—which meant that I could not devote the time I would have liked to other patients.

The last call of the day to me before she signed herself out of the hospital went something like: "You f . . . bitch, you made up the whole story to protect your f . . . nurses. I'll take you all to the press, so the world will know how fake you are and how you frame innocent people!" After she hung up, I contacted her family physician again, whom I had kept informed regarding Neda's behaviour, to make sure he didn't renew Neda's Demerol supply at home. Unfortunately, this doctor was young and rather gullible, and he had actually helped Neda store large quantities of the injectable narcotics and sedating drugs at home, which her dutiful husband would bring into the hospital. I wrote a detailed report of everything that happened with Neda in case she ever complained about me to the College of Physicians and Surgeons of Ontario.

After her discharge from the hospital, Neda kept phoning daily. The worker at our public relations office had a hard time holding her tongue and not reciprocating the cascade of verbal abuse to which she was submitted daily, and so did I. But finally, I lost it and told Neda that next time she called I would phone the police. I guess it worked—in fact, maybe I should have lost it earlier—because finally Neda stopped calling and left me alone. Subsequently, her family physician referred her to a detoxification centre.

Doctors who treat patients in pain frequently encounter people who are, to put it mildly, not always personable, and I have had my share—patients who can be litigious, neurotic, psychotic, verbally abusive, unreasonably demanding, expectant of special favours, non-compliant, stubborn or self-diagnosing (without any particular expertise). Chronic intractable pain will lead the hardest patients and pain problems to pain clinics, unlike the patients a typical family physician usually sees.

Am I complaining? Maybe a little, as things get tough some days—but it would be wrong to suggest that I lead a life of misery, and that the majority of my patients are personally troublesome. It is all the other patients, the hundreds and the thousands, who keep my flame lit.

I still fondly remember Yien Ho, for example, who was referred to me about two decades ago by the Workers' Compensation Board. His right thumb had been caught in a machine in the meat factory where he worked. Soon after, the thumb had to be amputated and Yien Ho was left with a lot of pain in his right hand. He had "phantom limb pain" exactly where the missing digit was supposed to be. But when he was admitted to my unit, my team soon realized that his actual problem was much greater than the one caused by his phantom thumb. Yien Ho was suffering from intense post-traumatic stress disorder.

A year after the accident, he still had vivid nightmares related to machines "eating up" his fingers, and would wake up drenched in sweat. He was afraid to go close to machines, and at times during the day he would revisit the accident in his mind. He was also quite depressed. But that was not all. I found out that he also had another very serious pain, in his heart.

Yien Ho was a "boat person." He had escaped from Cambodia with many others some years before and found his way to Canada. In his homeland, he had been an established businessman and landowner. But in Toronto, he became a factory worker. Just over 50, with little English, he followed the fate of thousands of other immigrants whose social status took a tumble in the transition from the old country to the new. I had started Yien Ho on analgesics and certain neuropathic medications, but he was making no great progress. His severe pain resisted all my treatments. As he was coming to see me often to adjust his drugs, he began gradually to engage in some conversation with me. One day as we were talking about him getting retrained in another job, I asked, "What would you like to do?"

"I have a dream," Yien Ho replied. "I wish I can wear a three-piece suit again!"

We discussed different jobs, one of which was real estate agent. Yien Ho knew that he needed to improve his English if he wanted to obtain a white-collar position. I wrote to the Workers' Compensation Board, which agreed to pay for him to upgrade his English and attend a real estate course, which, if he passed, would grant him his licence. Two years went by between upgrading his English and going through the course. Yien Ho struggled, but to his credit he asked to take his exams twice to make sure he scored the highest possible marks. During his regular visits, he would tell me how hard he was studying, and most of the time we ended up talking more about the course and the real estate market than his pain. Nevertheless, I encouraged him and told him that I strongly believe that if one perseveres, the sky is the limit.

Then Yien Ho disappeared from my practice for about six months. One day, he knocked at my door unexpectedly. To my surprise, he was dressed in a dark, three-piece suit and a matching tie. His face was glowing and he was holding a big package in his hands.

"Good heavens, where have you been?" I asked.

"Well" he said slowly, with clear but accented English, "I got my real estate licence and I sold my first house. This gift is for you. I paid for it from that sale, you know."

Yien Ho carefully peeled the wrapping paper and the supporting carton away. He unveiled a large, elaborate golden frame. Behind the glass there were a few sentences engraved in a Chinese dialect, but no picture.

"What does it say?" I asked curiously.

"I went to a special artist and I told him what to write. So it says here that you are 'not only a good doctor for bodies but also for souls.' You helped me reach my dream. Did you notice I wear a suit today?"

"Not only did I see it, but you also look pretty good," I replied.

When Yien Ho left he had a smile, and I was hiding my misty eyes. I never saw him again. But the golden frame has followed me from office to office, whenever my program has moved, a constant reminder of the indomitable human spirit.

Roy was a policeman in a region just outside Toronto. While alone driving his cruiser about 12 years ago, he responded to a call from the Ontario Provincial Police (OPP), who were in pursuit of a fellow who was on a shooting rampage on Highway 401, the main expressway through the most populated part of Ontario. The OPP set up a barricade under a bridge to stop the suspect, but could not tell Roy because his communication system was not working. The suspect smashed his car on the barricade and so did Roy, whom I saw about one and a half to two years after the accident. Roy didn't break any bones in the crash, but he was badly bruised. I learned there was a special insurance policy on the police cruiser Roy was driving. The OPP used the money to replace the cruiser, but Roy's injuries fell under the Workers' Compensation Board. By the time he was referred to me, Roy had a deep ache in his left chest wall, going down his whole left arm and hand, with pins and needles sensation in the last two fingers of the hand. He was told he had suffered only soft tissue injuries and he was supposed to have recovered long ago. But he hadn't, so the natural route was my pain clinic.

When I examined him, Roy proved to be a muscular man in his early 30s. He had a wife (on the same police force) and two kids. To make a long story short, I discovered that Roy had thoracic outlet syndrome. This is a clinical disorder in which the so-called neurovascular bundle of the arm (the artery, the vein and the brachial plexus) providing blood and innervation to the arm was somehow squeezed in a narrow space at the web of the neck, between the collar bone and the first rib. My tests actually showed a tremendous degree of obstruction in the vein and the artery. We had no choice but to operate on Roy. During the surgery, the surgeon found extensive scar tissue that was responsible for choking the neurovascular bundle. The adhesions (scarring) had resulted from a rupture of the muscles around the bundle during the accident. The surgery performed on Roy was unfortunately not that great a success. The scar tissue had been there for too long before the surgery and some permanent damage had been done. Roy continued to suffer with arm pain that I tried to manage with medications and therapy.

But beyond the physical pain, Roy was suffering greatly with emotional pain. No medicine or surgery could heal his battered dignity, as his police division was unable and unwilling to accommodate his disability. Roy could not be out in the street anymore. But he was a computer wizard and his skills could—and I believe should—have been used in an office position. The story was more complex than I thought. Prior to Roy's injury, he had had a falling out with his division over something he felt it was doing wrong. So when he got injured, there was no great effort to assist him in returning to work. Roy was "reduced to bringing the coffee to the office," as he later alleged in a human rights violation suit, several hundred pages long, that he initiated 10 years after his injury. Meanwhile, when his sick days per year were exhausted, he would go for months without pay, as workers' compensation was slow to kick in. There were two or three Christmases that he took his TV to the pawnbroker so he could buy food for the house. His marriage was falling apart, as his wife could not cope with him and his pain, the reduced income and the gossip at work.

I remember one particular instance when I had to be involved. Roy was without money again. I approached the Attorney General's office (at that time Ontario had a socialist New Democratic Party [NDP] government). I wrote a scathing letter, telling them how ironic it was that the police had money from the insurance to repair the cruiser but no money in the system to repair the human being. I got a call from the Attorney General's office and I was assured they were going to look into the case very quickly on humanitarian grounds. A month later, nobody had talked to me and nothing had been done with Roy and his police division. So, I called again, reaching the same fellow who had talked to me before.

"I am sorry," I said "but I am dealing with a very difficult situation. I have been approached by the press (I gave some name) about this case and I do not really know what to say. Of course, I am a supporter of the government and I do not want to have this making news and smearing the government's reputation." That I was an NDP supporter was true, but what I said about the press waiting to speak to me was a lie. My lie worked. Roy's payment was reinstated within days. (The arrangement unfortunately fell apart a year later, when the government changed.)

Roy went on to launch his human rights suit. It took years, a lot of pain and a tremendous amount of stress. In the process Roy came to see me, alarmed. His medications were not working; he needed a lot more as his pain had become excruciating. He said, also, that he was developing diffuse numbness throughout the left side of his body that was worrying him very much. Unfortunately, by the time I examined him, Roy had lost a good deal of sensation from the whole left side of the body, exactly the type of sensory deficit described in Chapter ten. His brain, under emotional duress, was playing terrible games.

I explained the whole thing to him. "Listen," I said. "Try to settle this as quickly as you can. You are under tremendous stress and your brain has given you signals. At some point, what you have now will be permanently engraved."

I cannot say, however, that Roy settled his case just because I told him to do so. A year or so later, an article about Roy by a sympathetic journalist appeared in one of the big daily newspapers. This probably sped up the process—and the closure—with the police division. Roy showed up glowing in my office a few months after the write-up. He had just settled his case with the police. He was a new man.

"You cannot imagine the weight that has been lifted off my chest. I am paying off my mortgage. I am setting up a home office and I am now looking at a couple of offers I have for an advisory role in human rights violation cases. I will not depend on workers' compensation again to feed my family. I can go on with my life."

Today, a black, engraved plaque from Roy's police union decorates another one of my walls, in recognition of what they perceived as my support for Roy.

John was a well-known and talented artist, film director and an accomplished painter. At 45, he had just gotten married to his beautiful wife Kathleen (this was John's second marriage). Life looked good, until the morning his car was run over by a Mack truck. John had to be extricated by the "Jaws of Life" and spent a month in the intensive care unit in a coma. He suffered major medical complications, including what we call adult respiratory distress syndrome, which damaged the lining of his lungs a great deal, leaving him with serious breathing problems. He was sent to me a year later because during the lengthy coma his peroneal nerve in both legs had been damaged. The peroneal nerve runs around the outer part of the leg and can be damaged if someone lies on the outside of the leg for a long time, which is exactly what happened to John during his coma. John could put up with everything—his difficult breathing, his problematic short memory (as he had suffered a brain injury as well) and the loss of his film career. But he could not put up with the severe burning shooting pain in both legs, so serious that he could not stand long enough to paint.

I tried different medications. A combination of morphine and a special neuropathic medication worked well. A year later, John brought me a large painting of a bellhop waiting for the elevator to arrive (one of the first works he painted once he could stand long enough), which today hangs prominently behind my chair. As I'm writing this, he has set up his studio, has a government grant to paint and a couple of commissioned pieces of art. Soon he will launch a show and he has invited me to attend.

Dave fell off the platform of his truck in 1984, at the age of 40, landing on both feet. He crushed his heels and a backbone. He ended up having six operations on his feet. Four years later, when he was referred to me, he had returned to work for a few hours every day; he was performing only light duties but he was in terrible pain. While most patients are referred to me by their family doctors, Dave was sent to me by his wife, a nurse, who called my secretary, Anna, and begged her for an appointment. Since he had returned to work, Dave had lost 11 kilograms (25 pounds). He was depressed and was swallowing over-the-counter pain medications like candies, as he seemed to be in terrific pain with his back and his feet. A proud man, he told me he had only one goal: to remain at work.

"Could you help me?" he asked.

"I'll try."

I put Dave on analgesics around the clock, rather than having him take them at the peak of his pain. I also gave him an antidepressant to help his sleep, mood and pain, and I sent him to our anesthetists for a special set of injections in his lower back, called "facet joint blocks." Today, 15 years later, Dave has remained at full-time work with the parks department of a local municipality. He drives a snowplow in the winter and a forklift in the summer. He has never taken a sick day off work, aside from a two-week leave three years ago, when he had another surgery in his right foot because of profound degenerative changes (arthritis). I see him regularly every six months and we almost never talk about the pain. But I know everything about his daughter, what she did at high school, which college she goes to now and what job opportunities she has. Dave tells me he owes it to me the fact that he stayed at work when everybody else was telling him to go on permanent disability. But I do not think so. It is the fire in his own belly, it is his own desire and indomitable spirit he should be grateful to, not me. If I did anything at all, other than medically, to take him beyond pain, it may be that I helped him find out what he had inside that could carry him through. Certainly, I do not mind seeing him regularly, if only to be able to use his story, which I tell to so many other patients who ask me if they will get better. I am sure they can with just a touch of help.

Lisa was only 24, with blue eyes, blonde hair, and a stunning face, when she tripped over a box and injured her left knee. I saw her two years after the injury, after she had made the rounds of many doctors, suffering from severe knee pain but gaining no diagnosis. Unfortunately, I found out she had developed reflex sympathetic dystrophy, the neuropathic pain syndrome discussed in Chapter five. Lisa tried every treatment I knew at the time, including medications, injections and surgery, each one failing to help. Lisa had a genetic marker that made her resistant to treatment, something I found out about in a study I did with one of my colleagues back in 1994 (described in Chapter two).[2] At that time, we interpreted this pilot study as showing that white women who develop this syndrome and do not get better seemed to possess some abnormal gene on chromosome 6, even if we could not tell exactly where.

But Lisa had decided she had a life to live, defective gene or otherwise. She changed her diet and her lifestyle, and several of the side effects of the drugs went away. To her surprise, her pain did not grow more serious. My medications, on the other hand, were doing her more harm than good. So she decided to drop almost all of them. And then she got married, registered in a part-time interior design course and finally she became pregnant. During pregnancy, her leg pain improved substantially because of her hormonal changes.

Meanwhile, I had bought a small, dilapidated house and I needed help with renovation ideas. I called her. "Would you take this as a project?" I asked. I could not afford to pay much, coming fresh from a divorce that nearly led me to bankruptcy, and she was a student who needed the project for her portfolio and charged little. It was a good deal for both of us.

Lisa ended up getting herself into a megaproject. Instead of little cosmetic changes, I decided to bite the bullet and borrow money to revamp the house from top to bottom, retaining only the walls. Lisa worked every day, sourcing paints, window dressings, appliances and so on, sometimes from her home, sometimes from mine. She was at the renovation site several times a week arranging things and supervising the various carpenters, kitchen installers and other workers. She became my right hand, and I hardly ever needed to take time off work to supervise the renovations. Lisa was there instead of me, but always leaning on her cane, with a purplish knee that she avoided touching. From time to time a frown on her beautiful face would show me some of her pain. But she never let life go. She had and still has a significant medical problem and lives with pain on a daily basis. However, she is now the wonderful mother of two robust boys and a loving wife and friend to her husband. And more than this, she has become a close friend of mine. Again, Lisa's story is one that I often recount to patients who I see are like her. She is someone who lives in chronic pain but still owns and controls her life instead of letting pain and suffering control her.

I strongly believe, and share my belief with my patients, that my skills and the skills of other pain doctors are merely helpers. I do not fix anyone. I lack the ability to perform miracles. I am only a partner in my patients' care, providing them with information, my knowledge and my experience. Beyond that, they really do the job themselves. To live with chronic pain means living with limitations. People with chronic pain often can no longer do what they used to do, but life is still beautiful and worth living if one can accept limitations and work around them.

Many patients who come to me are upset about their loss and their problem. I try to encourage them to think of the abilities and functions they still have and not what they lost. I also advise them that smaller problems fade away when we are faced with bigger troubles, and I use the following story to help them understand my viewpoint.

Once, a young man attended a wise man's lecture. At the end, he felt very hopeful that the wise man would help him with his problem.

"Sir," he said, "I have a serious problem and I need your help."

"Certainly," the wise man replied. "I'll tell you right now how to fix it."

"But sir," the young man protested, "I have not even told you what my problem is. How are you going to help me fix it?"

"Son, I do not need to know your problem. Just go out there, find someone with a bigger problem and yours will be solved on its own!"

Twelve

THE POLITICS OF PAIN

Anyone who has suffered chronic pain knows that pain is serious. But I'm sure, as well, that anyone who has worked in the field of chronic pain as I have knows that it has not always been taken seriously enough, at least until lately. I believe that my own experience is illustrative, when I look back at the energy and resources that have been required just to ensure that my program could make it as a viable centre for pain treatment and research.

When I founded my program 20 years ago at the Toronto Western Hospital (a teaching hospital affiliated with the University of Toronto), to ensure its survival, both my assistant, Anna, and I worked 12-hour days so we could see enough patients. For five years I never took a day off. I was on call seven days a week, 24 hours a day. I gave birth in a hurry to two children: my eldest, Nicholas, arrived prematurely when my water broke six weeks before his due date, while working in the laboratory on my master's thesis. Seventeen months later, my younger son, Alex, was induced close to his due date, since he had decided to rest his head inside my pelvis on my obturator nerve—the one that works the adductor muscles and the inner thigh—giving me horrendous leg spasms. After both deliveries I was back at work parttime in 10 days and fulltime in 30 days. In those days, female doctors like me did not have any privileges whatsoever for maternity leave or compensation, in contrast to what medical women enjoy today in my own hospital and the University of Toronto. Despite the fact that chronic pain even then was a widespread problem, it elicited no sympathy from governments, hospital administrators or even the medical establishment. I did not want to risk closure of my unit during a prolonged absence (as there was no one to replace me during potential leave or sickness).

As a territory to study in the beginning of my career, pain was no man's land—and no woman's either. My job was akin to what they call in the want ads a "person Friday"—a sort of "fixer" who could bring together all the people who looked after the various aspects of chronic pain—neurosurgeons, anaesthetists, psychiatrists, psychologists and other health care workers. It was up to me to assemble these specialists and create some kind of multidisciplinary program. This meant that I had the punishing workload of a resident (trainee doctor) and all the heavy responsibilities of a staff doctor. I had been given six beds for chronic pain patients while at the same time I was running an outpatient clinic a few days a week. Yet the clinical work was not my only chore. I was also supposed to be spending nearly all of my time in research, as I had registered with the Institute of Medical Science at the University of Toronto for my master's degree.

In those years I was never sure that my program was going to survive. Chronic pain practice based on the Canadian fee-for-service system makes no allowance for a living that is commensurate with the amount of work involved. Nor does the system make it easy for doctors to do a thorough job with patients who require a tremendous amount of time and care given the complexity of their problems. Chronic pain is labour-intensive, non-remunerative compared with other disciplines and unglamorous—"unsexy," as I have been heard complaining for many years now. In the 1980s, a double lung and heart transplant costing a quarter of a million dollars for one patient would make newspaper headlines, while chronic pain affecting a large percentage of the population was not impressive enough to occupy even a quarter of a page in the middle section of a newspaper, except on rare occasions.

However, I remember with everlasting gratitude a few people along my way to whom I owe unequivocally the existence and survival of my program. These people saved us from potential extinction in crucial periods. The first one is a woman who was then a member of the board of trustees of the Toronto Western Hospital. (The hospital subsequently merged with the Toronto General Hospital and Princess Margaret Hospital, to become what we know today as the University Health Network in Toronto, with three individual sites.) This woman was introduced to me by my professor of physical medicine in the mid-1980s. She took a liking to me (and the subject of chronic pain) because she knew pain firsthand: she had suffered for years with serious pain until finally the cause was found. She and some of her friends raised enough funds to allow me to hire a doctor trainee (fellow) to assist me with my workload in the clinic—this kept my program and me from collapse. She also generously funded our first computer and laser printer. Her generosity carried my research and the clinical activities of my program for a few years.

Nevertheless, at the beginning of 1990, I met with one of the most serious crises my program and I had faced. The department of medicine I belonged to was changing its financial rules for the member doctors. When I was asked to increase my productivity by 40 per cent I realized I was already working beyond capacity. My day had no more hours. I was preparing to hand in my resignation and close down the program. But then some kind of miracle happened.

A patient of mine who subsequently became wheelchair-bound could not come and see me any more, for the simple reason that the building where my office was located was not wheelchair accessible. Her husband, who like her was in his 70s, grateful for the care his wife was receiving, visited the Ontario Ministry of Health several times and also called daily, asking if there was anything that could be done to help my program acquire better facilities. Apparently, tired of the persistent old man, the provincial bureaucrats put him in contact with a small branch of the Ontario Ministry of Health, called the Alternative Payment Program. This branch was dealing with programs and doctors who had given up their fee-for-service method of payment through the Ontario Health Insurance Plan, my province's publicly funded health care program, in exchange for a fixed salary. This method of remuneration is common in many parts of the world where medical care is publicly funded, but it was rarely used in Ontario then. The Alternative Payment Program's manager offered to help me. On my own, I entered negotiations with the government.

But nothing was ever easy for my program and me. The negotiations progressed to formulating a draft contract, but then a disaster occurred. To the best of my knowledge, this was the first time ever that the Toronto Western Hospital was running a large deficit, and the administrators decided that the way to save money was to cut down on beds. They told all the members of the department of medicine that there would be a 10 per cent across-the-board reduction in beds. I soon realized that they meant a 10 per cent reduction for the "worthwhile" programs, but a much greater bed loss for the ones deemed insignificant by the administrators—such as my program. The morning after the announcement I woke up to find *all* of my six beds gone.

I was in despair. The government contract was contingent upon my maintaining both an outpatient and an in-patient facility. I turned to the Medical Advisory Committee, a senior body of doctors that deals with administrative hospital matters. Twenty-four hours later, the chairman, "Dr. M.," walked into my cramped office to tell me "how sorry he was, but there was nothing that could be done." I had anticipated such an answer, and I had already done my homework.

"You have seen my guns but you have not seen my bazookas yet!" I told him.

"What do you mean?" the doctor asked in panic, perhaps misconstruing the meaning of my threat.

What I meant to convey was that I had been a politically active student during the turbulent years of junta dictatorship in Greece (from 1967 to 1974), and I had learned some hard lessons, which equipped me with fighting skills that could be applied to everyday life if necessary. Now I was determined to put these skills to good use in Canada, too.

I had anticipated that my own hospital administrators and colleagues would meet the threat of our clinic's closure with inertia and indifference. Meanwhile, though, I had been in contact with a wonderful woman, Diane Kent, who was the founder and president of a patient support group called the Ontario Chapter of the North American Chronic Pain Association. Diane was suffering from failed back syndrome and had been my patient for years. "Don't worry," she assured me, "we will be there for the program, as you have been there for us."

Diane waited for my call while she lined up a long list of pain patients prepared to hit the phones and meet the press.

"For goodness' sake," Dr. M. said. "Don't do this. At least speak to the hospital president first."

I was expecting nothing good to come of this, but I bent and got on the phone with the hospital president. I was right again. The president (who must have had a very bad day) chewed me out: "You said you are in negotiations with the government to fund you? If they have money to fund you, then they had better cover my hospital deficit too. No beds. You will just have to operate on an outpatient basis."

That would have been disastrous. The government was not going to finalize my contract, while my unit would be severely limited in the kinds of investigations and treatment we could offer to people in pain. I huffed: "Well sir, I can assure you, if there are no beds, there will be no outpatient program either."

"Who says so?" the president asked.

"I do, sir. I founded the program and have poured my blood and soul into it. If it can't be the best, it better not be at all." I could almost feel the force as he crashed down the phone on the cradle. I dialled Diane's number.

It was Friday afternoon. Within 48 hours the hospital's public relations department had received at least 50 calls from irate patients. On Monday morning, a few of the patients were waiting outside the president's office. By Monday afternoon, an urgent meeting had been set up for the heads of the respective departments (who had contributed beds to my program) to meet and "see what could be done with the pain clinic's beds." But there was a problem: Although I was founder and director of the program, I had not been invited to the meeting! I ran to the office of the then physician-in-chief, Dr. Arnie Aberman (who later became the dean of Medicine at the University of Toronto). Arnie was vocally proclaiming his support for professional women.

"Well, Arnie, put your money where your mouth is. You cannot go to this meeting without me."

Arnie consoled me. "Don't worry," he said. "You will be there. But for goodness' sake, Angela, just take a book, pretend you are studying and let me negotiate for you!" Arnie Aberman was probably right. I was angry—so angry that my head was hot. And hot heads can say stupid things sometimes. So, I took

Arnie's advice and behaved with restraint. It wasn't easy. The president was steaming as he explained to the chiefs how much trouble my patients and I had given him. Nevertheless, by the end of the day, thanks to Arnie's negotiating skills, I had most of my beds back. I signed my government contract and to this date, 13 years later, my little program is still alive and well (despite other mishaps and troubles that we had over the years).

To me, the story of my battle to keep my pain program alive offers a lot of lessons—about politics, about the struggle for health care dollars and about the changing perception among professionals and the public of pain, pain research and pain relief. It is telling that once my contract was signed and sealed, the president of the hospital met me at a professional gathering and congratulated me with a warm handshake, as if we were old friends. Then he turned around and offered my program a new space . . . 10 times larger than the little basement cubbyhole I had been using! How could I refuse?

As of November 2001, 19 years after the inception of the program and after several more moves, my pain clinic has its own premises at last. Our quarters are neither large nor luxurious, but at least we have a permanent home under the umbrella of the prestigious Neuroscience Group at the Toronto Western Hospital. Chronic pain is finally recognized at my own hospital.

Chronic Pain in Canada

The 1990s saw a lot of changes in chronic pain care, but these changes didn't happen accidentally. Chronic pain became an important issue in Ontario when big bucks began to be invested in treatment—an investment that was the product of changes in automobile insurance in the province.

There are two categories of automobile insurance. One is based on the tort system, in which the two parties go to court and the party found at fault for the car accident has to award damages to the other party (usually through his or her insurer). The other type of compensation is through no-fault insurance (which for most accidents replaced the tort system in Ontario in 1990). In this system the insured's own company pays, regardless of who is at fault. This removes the need for costly and time-consuming court battles over liability. Someone injured in an accident can still sue for damages, but only if an "injury threshold" has been reached. This threshold requires that there be "permanent and serious impairment of an important bodily function caused by an injury which was physical in nature." To ensure that only the most serious injuries would lead to arguments in court over liability, spending on medical care and rehabilitation of accident victims increased rather generously.

Within a few years of the establishment of no-fault insurance in Ontario, Designated Assessment Centres (DACs) for determination of the victim's rehabilitation needs sprang up across the province. Naturally, these DACs deal with the single most important complaint of accident victims—pain. In 1988, a survey of all Canadian facilities or pain programs counted 37 pain clinics throughout the country, with 60 per cent of them in Ontario and Quebec.[1] Nearly a decade later, I found to my surprise how much things had changed in Ontario. In 1997, I was running for chair of the Chronic Pain Section of the Ontario Medical Association, and I had to fax my goals and objectives and those of my team to all the clinics where physicians worked with pain patients. I discovered to my astonishment that there were more than 300 pain clinics (most of them DACs) in Ontario alone—more than a tenfold increase in less than 10 years. These clinics specialize in assessing and treating pain, particularly pain arising from motor vehicle accident injuries. What had been a lonely practice was now a big business in the medicolegal world, and an expensive one too.

No-fault insurance shaped the way pain was viewed in Ontario. Inevitably, changes came to regulatory policies and in the policies of disability and compensation carriers. Around 1996, the College of Physicians and Surgeons of Ontario (CPSO) recognized that chronic pain management is a significant issue for practising physicians. To educate the province's doctors, the CPSO created a Chronic Pain Task Force (which I co-chaired) to provide guidelines for the medical management of chronic non-malignant pain as I discussed in Chapter eight. The guidelines were formulated based on a consolidated review of the best literature in chronic pain and a summary of what had been found through research to work or not work. For the first time, doctors in Ontario had a medical roadmap to help them manage chronic pain. These guidelines quickly became the most sought-after publication of the CPSO, so I, among others, am now responsible for updating them with the newest medical information every few years.

Around the same time, the Workers' Compensation Board of Ontario called in a team of experts to help redefine its policies on chronic pain and chronic pain–related disability. This expert panel reviewed the existing literature and produced treatment recommendations, which in many ways mirror those produced by our group under the CPSO mandate. Unfortunately, the work of the panel supported the concept of dualism of pain, as chronic pain was viewed as either physical or psychological.

On another front, the University of Toronto assisted in the creation of the University of Toronto Centre for the Study of Pain (UTCSP). The centre is a "virtual reality" establishment, based in Toronto, that unites health professionals and scientists in the city working in pain management, education and research. It was inaugurated during the ninth World Congress in Pain in Vienna in 1999. Several clinicians and scientists, including me, served as founding members of the centre. Today, UTCSP has started attracting world-renowned scientists, who have decided to make Toronto their home.

Pain has been recognized now as an important health issue in many provinces beyond Ontario, as similar moves for bringing together those working in the pain field take place across Canada. Academic centres are collaborating to form a National Centre of Excellence to link clinicians and scientists, so we can understand and manage pain more effectively. In addition, the Canadian Pain Society, an association of clinicians and scientists working in the area of pain, has been very active in enhancing awareness and bringing changes in the management of pain to the public and administrators.

All this means a lot to me as a professional. Where I live and practise, pain now has a face—it is a recognized discipline, and millions of dollars have been allocated to its study and treatment in the last decade. But this is only the tip of the iceberg, as many more millions are needed. Where once it was a vague ailment—often little more than a grab bag of complaints and suggestions for relief—pain is now considered a significant health issue and its social and economic consequences are taken more seriously.

As well, the pharmaceutical industry has become substantially involved in chronic pain. The industry's emphasis is exclusively geared toward the biomedical aspects of pain, as their profits are made from developing and selling drugs. In my view, the industry's interest is a double-edged sword. Megadollars devoted to development of new drugs will undoubtedly help new discoveries and better pain understanding and management. On the other hand, pouring substantial amounts of money into the support and promotion of the biomedical aspects of pain exclusively may undermine the need for more comprehensive pain management that takes into account both biomedical and psychological/psychosocial factors.

There is a plethora of pain references in the media nowadays. Newspapers and magazines, radio and television shows talk about pain in the young and old, acute pain after surgery, cancer pain and chronic non-cancer pain. Doctors, educators, administrators, policy-makers, insurers and the public are paying attention to a lot of the chatter too. Pain clinics, once treated as medical stepchildren, now open up in prestigious teaching and community hospitals. Administrators are more interested in providing care to patients with pain. Even my own hospital declared pain "a priority" in 2002.

What a change! Twenty years after the creation of my small pain program, pain is "hot." In the U.S., just before the end of his presidency, Bill Clinton declared the first 10 years of the twenty-first century as the "Decade of Pain Awareness and Research." American hospitals are now officially bound to chart pain "as the fifth vital sign" (after pulse, breathing, blood pressure and temperature), following the successful efforts of the Joint Committee on Accreditation of Healthcare Organizations, which identified pain programs and began to track patients' treatment. All of us are now better aware of the reality of untreated, undertreated, overtreated and misdiagnosed pain and its impact on human suffering as well as our collective wallet.

Awareness, however, has implications.

The Chronic Pain Epidemic

When James, in his mid-30s, was wheeled into my office some years ago, he looked as if he had suffered a stroke or some kind of brain injury. He was sitting in a wheelchair, head tilted to the right, left arm resting on his lap, speaking slowly as if his tongue were stuck in his mouth, having great difficulty expressing himself. At times his face would twitch or he would drool from the corner of his mouth. To my surprise I learned that he had not suffered a stroke; he had simply been involved in a minor car accident four years before. The accident seemed straightforward and unremarkable. James had been the driver, approaching a stop sign, when he was rear-ended by another car at minimal speed. He got out of the car immediately, realized it was a minor fender-bender, exchanged his particulars with the other driver and drove home. There were no police involved, no ambulance and not much pain either. The next morning, he had a bit of a stiff neck. By the afternoon, though, his pain spread to his upper back. He saw his family practitioner the next day and by that time, he felt forgetful and confused.

The family doctor diagnosed whiplash and lumbar sprain and sent him for physiotherapy. So James did not go to work but instead to intense therapy, paid for by the insurance company, nearly every day. One day, when he looked slightly forgetful, a zealous therapist wondered if James had suffered a head injury, even though James hadn't banged his head or felt dazed during or just after the accident. She let James and his physician know about her concerns. Shortly after, James and his wife consulted a lawyer, and additional rehabilitation services were mobilized. James started attending Designated Assessment Centres for repeated assessments, but he nevertheless became sicker and sicker.

He was referred to a program dealing with "acquired brain injury." This term means brain damage that is believed by some to have been caused by some kind of jolting event, even one as small as the fender-bender in which James hadn't hit his head. I'm afraid that I have seen proponents of acquired brain damage of this sort diagnose "damaged brains" after the impact of forces similar to a strong sneeze. A late colleague of mine, Ann Taylor, used to joke, "Imagine how many 'brain-dead' people would go around after a good cold!" Nevertheless, once he was in the "acquired brain damage" program, James was taught all his limitations, plus many more than he could ever imagine himself.

By the time James was referred to me, he used a wheelchair for any activity outside the house, he needed help for personal hygiene and feeding, he could hardly walk a couple of steps and even then only with the help of canes, his speech was slurred, he had diffuse pains all over, his left side was weak and he was terribly forgetful and confused. He had a long list of diagnoses all furnished to him by well-meaning physicians and zealous health professionals such as chiropractors, physiotherapists and kinesiologists: post-traumatic headaches, post-concussion syndrome, closed head injury, fibromyalgia, dizziness due to inner ear damage, occipital neuralgia, cervicogenic headaches, cervical facet joint syndrome, lumbar facet joint syndrome, temporomandibular joint disorder, shoulder tendonitis and more. James had home care services, including a physiotherapist, an occupational therapist and a nurse. He simply could not take care of himself, let alone his two young kids, and his wife worked part time to support the family.

I decided to admit him. I strongly suspected that what I was seeing in James was nothing more than a "conversion reaction," a psychological condition in which patients transform intolerable stresses or uncomfortable emotions into physical symptoms. I decided to give him an intravenous injection of normal saline (sterile water), explaining that it would be followed by some other drug as is customary in my unit. James seemed hopeful that we were going to help him. After all, he was coming to a highly reputed pain clinic in the big city. As soon as the first few drops of saline entered his system, James's pain started to drop precipitously. His strength started returning, his head straightened up, his left elbow unfolded, and he managed to get out of the bed by himself. He walked back and forth the length of the room, slowly but unaided. After this, a few drops of a medium-action barbiturate wiped away the last traces of his pain.

James had not felt such complete relief in four years. He became euphoric, giggling happily and pacing the floor swiftly. My colleagues in psychiatry and psychology confirmed that indeed he had the type of personality that would not cope well with stress and that tended to express feelings or pressures with body symptoms. James walked out of my unit four days later pushing the wheelchair, instead of being rolled out by his wife.

Unfortunately, the effects lasted only one week. Our team pleaded urgently with James's doctor, with a copy of our correspondence sent to his lawyer, to stop "medicalizing" James's problems. We thought he should be enrolled instead in an intensive cognitive-behavioural psychosocial rehabilitation program. But our advice was not followed. I heard from his wife a month later. By then, not only was James back in his wheelchair, now even inside the house, but he had developed new symptoms, including shaking hands and twisting movements of his head. He could swallow only liquids. And he had trouble communicating.

His rehabilitation counsellor urgently dispatched a speech therapist to study his swallowing problem and to teach him how to speak.

The moral of James's story is that a minor sprain in a minor car accident was blown up to a major issue in terms of James's own perception of what happened to him and in terms of the ideas planted in his head by the many professionals he saw. Why? In the first place his personality fabric was such that emotional stressors were converted into physical symptoms. Second, he believed what he had been told: that the accident probably shook up and damaged his brain plus several other parts of his body, including his cervical and lumbar spine, his jaws and his ears. Simple, unsophisticated and hyper-suggestible, James learned many symptoms or even developed new ones, week after week, particularly after participating in the "acquired brain injury" program. Petrified that his brain was all smashed up, James and his wife worried about their future. His keen lawyer, despite good intentions, contributed to James's malady by channelling him to numerous medical experts and other zealous health care providers who diagnosed multiple physical entities. James took all this in. He became the victim of his own personality, his fate the captive of his doctors, health care providers and lawyers.

James, as well as numerous others like him whom I have seen over the past 20 years, is an example of sufferers from a new breed of disorders that have invaded Western society in epidemic proportions. Disorders such as repetitive strain injury, fibromyalgia, temporomandibular disorders, chronic fatigue syndrome and myalgic encephalomyelitis, acquired brain injury, environmental supersensitivity and sick building syndrome, whiplash and non-specific low back pain complaints all appeared in the late twentieth century. In the nineteenth century, as industrialization spread, bizarre disorders had emerged in similar proportions, such as railway spine in Victorian England and neurasthenia in the United States. Most of these disorders are painful—the victims truly suffer—but besides pain, there are often a multitude of tangential symptoms that can be difficult to connect to the original complaint: mental confusion and forgetfulness, depression, anxiety, excessive fatigue, sleep disturbances, loss of sexual desire or impotence and so on. Today's disorders and their nineteenth-century cousins are similar in that both have triggered hundreds of research papers, led to billions of dollars in health care spending, disability payments and legal fees, a constant conflict between believers and non-believers in these disorders—professionals or otherwise—and, most importantly, they have created never-ending numbers of people whose lives have become lost to invalidism and chronic illnesses.

Some of these conditions became major causes of disability in industrialized nations, and then nearly vanished. Such an example is the repetitive strain injury (RSI) syndrome. Its rise and fall in Australia in the 1980s is extremely well documented.[2] For many years, repetitive movements in general have been a well known but not frequent cause of inflammation of tendon sheaths of the forearm, and had not caused chronic health problems.[3] When computers were first introduced in Australia, discomfort attributed to repetitive wrist movements was named RSI and considered a compensable disorder in the early 1980s. The disorder spread in the workplace like an epidemic. Numerous papers were written on the syndrome, thousands of patients were sent out of the workforce and the costs of disability and health care mounted.[4] However, by the mid-1980s it became apparent that social factors were much more prevalent than physical ones in the generation of the symptoms, and the disorder soon was nearly abandoned. The Australian government reduced compensation for the condition and the relationship between RSI and chronic pain was found by the courts to be unproven.[5]

In my view, other conditions, such as fibromyalgia and chronic fatigue syndrome, are diagnosed indiscriminately in large numbers of patients. This is *not* to say that many of these conditions do not exist, but that they are diagnosed much more frequently than they should be, and not infrequently the real cause of pain and disability is different from the one originally thought. Chronic painful illnesses must be viewed from the whole person's perspective instead of the biomedical or psychosocial perspective unilaterally.

Understanding such illnesses is analogous to the old cliché about the elephant and a bunch of blind men. One man touches the trunk and says the elephant feels like a rope, the other one touches the tail and thinks the elephant is like a snake and the third one touches the leg and says the elephants is like a tree. To understand what the entity really is, one must view not just the symptoms but the whole person. In other words, one needs to understand the way the person feels, how he or she functions in his world and the way he or she is influenced by his or her environment.

Let's take for example low back pain and its associated disabilities, as expressed in lost work days or money spent for compensation and health care. In statistical terms, low back pain in the workplace has risen to epidemic proportions in the industrialized world. At the same time, it continues to remain manageable in developing countries. Why the discrepancy? It does not seem to me that over the last century, back pain sufferers in Canada, the United States, Britain, Sweden, Australia and so on have developed a greater number of herniated discs or degenerated spines. Unquestionably, though, they take much more time off work, they utilize a much larger number of treatments and they become unemployed or disabled in frightening numbers at tremendous cost to society. As I discussed in Chapter six, among those who develop acute low back pain in the workplace, 10 per cent will end up with chronic low back pain and they will consume 80 per cent of the money spent to cover lost work days, permanent disability and health care costs. While changes in lifestyle (obesity, lack of exercise and general deconditioning due to sedentary occupations) may contribute to higher incidence of acute or recurrent low back pain, studies are concluding that persistent or chronic low back pain in the workplace is more linked with psychological or social factors than with physical ones.[6]

Risk factors for developing chronic low back pain in the workplace have much to do with a previous history of chronic pain; whether one likes one's job or not; the presence of depression, anxiety, and any kind of stress; and even the availability of compensation that may serve as a financial disincentive. The list of risk factors goes on and on, as chronic back pain may be perpetuated by the beliefs of both patients and health care providers, as well as vested interests and financial incentives for the providers to keep treating the low back pain victim.[7] I also strongly believe that what happens in one's life and how one responds to the different stresses may very well engrave biochemical and other changes in the neuronal circuits that control pain and perpetuate pain and disability.

For back pain and any other diseases of such epidemic proportions, I think it's important to look beyond the plain physical causes and our previously unquestioned assumptions about the role of trauma or injury. Back pain has been with us for thousands of years, but its ascent to epidemic proportion happened only in the last five decades. A host of factors aside from the physical ailment are important; we live in a society that often promotes invalidism through disease "templates" that guide us in how we are "supposed" to feel when we have chronic pain, and often through public policies (in terms of health care coverage and compensation) that can actually foster disability. While society's support for disability is important and necessary, at times it becomes a double-edged sword.

The influence of socio-economic and environmental factors is often so powerful that good science can at times become ineffective. For example, health care agencies in Canada, the United States and Britain have published practice guidelines for health care providers, drawn from scientific studies, on how to treat episodes of acute low back pain. The recommendations include conducting a thorough clinical examination to make sure one does not miss the rare ominous cause of low back pain, avoiding investigations like X-rays (unless a specific suspicion arises), recommending regular simple physical activities instead of lying down in bed, and discouraging the use of muscle relaxants and opioids. It has not been easy to persuade either physicians or patients to follow these recommendations, as societal perceptions and practitioners' interests play a much higher role than science in shaping decisions about treatment. In the U.S., the guidelines[8] caused so much anger within the medical establishment that doctors nearly convinced Congress to cancel the funding for the agency that produced them.[9]

Can the attitudes and beliefs of health care providers and patients change? And if so, what will it take? In Australia, Dr. Rachelle Buchbinder, a rheumatologist and epidemiologist, organized a media campaign to try to change peoples' beliefs regarding the management of low back pain. Her research earned her the prestigious Volvo Award for clinical studies in 2001.[10] Dr. Buchbinder's media program began in 1997 in the state of Victoria. The campaign advised patients with back pain to stay active, exercise and remain at work rather than rest for prolonged periods. The campaign used prime-time television commercials in which international and national medical experts and Australian sports and TV personalities talked about back pain, including their own, and how to manage it successfully, recommending the simple principles of activity and exercise over inertia. Radio and print ads, billboards, posters, public seminars, workplace visits and news articles augmented the TV campaign. An educational "Back Booklet" was made available widely and translated into 16 languages, and all the state's doctors received recommendations for pain management of employees hurt at work. Each advertisement was endorsed by a national professional organization, such as physicians, surgeons and chiropractors, and the campaign was supported by Australia's powerful labour unions. It was an undertaking of immense proportions and incredible logistics, but it was all done and completed successfully within three years, and the results were spectacular. Patients and doctors alike showed significant changes in attitude and beliefs toward low back pain. The number of workers who claimed a back injury dropped by 15 per cent, which was more than anticipated, saving 20 per cent of the medical costs that would have been incurred otherwise.

Unfortunately, the story does not end here. The campaign was funded by the Australian state's workers' compensation board; it cost $10 million (Australian) and saved more than six times what was spent. But when Dr. Buchbinder came to my own hospital in May 2002 and discussed the aftermath, it was less than encouraging. After the campaign had run for three years, the state government changed hands and the labour unions did an about-face on their previous support for the program. Instead of supporting the campaign, the new regime ordered an investigation of the researchers, alleging that there had been fraudulent use of research funds (all were completely exonerated). The labour movement as well took an adversarial position, launching its own publicity campaign depicting injured workers in wheelchairs due to "employer negligence" who "downplay" the workers' injuries and their back pain.

What happened in Victoria, Australia, confirms for me that when vested interests are at stake, science is under siege. I don't think that situation is unique. In Canada, Saskatchewan's government insurance program commissioned three reputable institutions to study the actual effects of the auto-insurance change from the tort to no-fault system. The study was sufficiently sound on a scientific basis and was published in the prestigious *New England Journal of Medicine*. It showed that after the switch to no-fault insurance, there was a 28 per cent drop in whiplash claims.[11] The lower number of claims was attributed to the fact that once compensation is not easily available, as in the case of no-fault insurance, those involved in minor motor vehicle accidents don't bother to file a claim and don't hire a lawyer. The study raised quite a bit of heated argument from those in the medical profession who believe that it does not accurately depict the true numbers of whiplash victims. It also raised the wrath of lawyers' associations. Dr. David Cassidy, the senior investigator of the study, came under attack by the *National Law Journal*,[12] the American Association of Trial Lawyers and others. Ultimately, accusations of fixing the results led the University of Saskatchewan to impound the research data and conduct an inquiry, only to conclude that the researchers were innocent and the study was indeed extremely well done from the scientific point of view. A change to no-fault insurance, minimizing tort claims, had saved the province of Saskatchewan, with one million residents, half a billion dollars in medical and legal costs over five years, even with, as mentioned earlier in this chapter, the increases in clinical treatment that no-fault regimes tend to bring. But the researchers who looked at the data and pointed to the impact of available compensation on the duration of disability were subjected to a barrage of personal and professional attacks, which they certainly did not expect.

My own experience with vested interests is relatively small, but I think it is significant. A few years ago, my team was interested in reviewing the complications of a popular procedure called sympathectomy, performed on patients with excessive sweating and certain kinds of pain. We ended up reviewing the worldwide literature for a total of 23,000 patients and 42,000 surgeries. The number and magnitude of complications that we discovered were astounding. When we published the results, I had several unpleasant communications with a certain group of doctors who perform the procedure frequently—the gist of their concern was that they were afraid our data would turn patients away and the U.S. insurance industry would refuse to pay the bills.[13]

When it comes to the politics of pain, I could write a second book full of stories. Over 20 years I think I have seen it all, with all the contrasts and contradictions—the bureaucracies and the bureaucrats; the legal system with both its strengths (gaining justice for pain sufferers) and its shortcomings (exploiting the system and prolonging the stress and costs); the backward-thinking workers' compensation regimes, which (at long last in Ontario), seem now to be trying to address the pain problem in all its magnitude; the devoted health care providers; the bandwagon jumpers; the pretend patients who try to milk the system; and, most of all, the genuine people in pain. It is this last group that keeps me going.

I know this group of pain sufferers—among them many of the individuals I describe in this book—also motivates a worldwide community of pain researchers, scientists and health care providers to keep doing what they do, to explore pain mechanisms and search for cures; to try to really understand what the sufferer is experiencing, on both a scientific level and on a personal level; and to translate our research findings into practical ways to prevent pain or help those in pain to feel better.

I believe in the Hippocratic Oath I took as a physician, and I also believe in the simple bit of advice I give my patients: "You must never give up hope until I do, and I never do."

EPILOGUE

One of the activities most important to me, aside from medicine and family life, is my involvement with martial arts. My encounters with tae kwon do, one of the ancient martial arts, have given me insights into human nature, myself and my ongoing discovery of what causes pain and how to respond to it.

By mid-1999, my tae kwon do master felt that I was ready to become a candidate for my first-degree black belt, a road that proved to be a tough one, as I needed many months of gruelling training. This meant that I would spend two hours in the gym nearly every day, always at the crack of dawn before I had to go to the office. This was in preparation for the horror of the "power weekend," a qualifying session that would determine whether I was ready to receive the black belt at a special ceremony a few weeks later.

I had been warned that the power weekend was set up to test our mettle—to deprive participants of sleep, to deplete every physical reserve, literally to bring us to our knees. It was meant to test all our limits. The only thing I could do to survive would be to cling to some sort of ephemeral spirit inside me, to keep alive the burning desire to make it through successfully. Unfortunately, my back pain started showing up from the beginning of the intense preparatory training. It was an ugly monster that I thought I had tamed . . . but I was wrong. The excessive demands of training and the abuse of my body had revived the sleeping villain. On some bad days I would freeze with acute, knife-like pains in the middle of a jump or a kick. Stretching, hot baths, a solid leather belt around my waist and lengthy warm-up periods let me break the pain cycle within half a day so I could pull through. Thank God, the pain would go away quickly; in the past it would last for weeks and months.

I finally made it to the weekend I feared so much, in May 2000. My group consisted of 10 candidates—seven adults between the ages of 37 and 52, and three children aged 9 to 12. All of us, including the children, had been training for several years. I calculated that in the 42 intense hours of that weekend, I had 20 hours of incessant training, four hours of sleep and about 2500 calories of liquid meal replacements. I also ran 10 kilometres (6 miles), climbed at least 1000 stairs, did 30 minutes of non-stop skipping and hundreds and hundreds of abdominal crunches and pushups—the "real" ones, on the palms or knuckles and the feet, not with knees on the floor. I and the rest of our group also performed several of our forms—a complex sequence of movements, each combination 20 to 40 movements long—one-step sparring, defence manoeuvres, movements to music and so on. For some of these I was blindfolded. For others I had a whole raw egg in my mouth—unco-ordinated breathing would crush the egg, but thank goodness I did all right. I also had to perform sequences of movements holding two cups half-filled with water in my outstretched fingers. Again, I managed not to spill the water on the floor, because each failure would be followed by punishment in the form of many crunches or knuckle pushups. To make matters worse, at some points each of the candidates had to face two attackers, all lean and mean first- and second-degree black belt instructors, many years younger than most of us. The fights were full contact, and while they each lasted for only a few minutes, we all felt as if they lasted for hours.

During this brutal weekend, lactic acid accumulation and tearing would ride through my muscles as I exceeded my personal threshold. After the first day of non-stop training I started becoming stiff and my flesh hurt with every move. But I managed to get through the ordeal and ignore most of the pain. During endurance-challenging tasks I would "tune myself out." On long runs, for example, I would fix my attention only on my two shoes as they pounded the pavement, ignoring my increasingly rigid and aching legs. During these "tuned-out" periods I could hear the instructors or the calls of the team, but they were very far away, even when they were physically close. I was not really "there"— I was living just for the moment. And despite what was happening to my body, I was feeling almost no pain.

Even when I had to participate in team tasks, I could still block my pain. I was able to refocus my attention to the task at hand, remain relatively unemotional, co-ordinate my moves and just do the job. But when I was between tasks, with my attention free to wander, all of a sudden, pain from my torn muscles would overwhelm me. It seemed to come from nowhere, hitting me as I would attempt to sit on the floor. It would last until the next task when, within moments, it would vanish again.

I made it through the power weekend. When I finally arrived home, I was at the point of complete mental and physical exhaustion. Then, a couple of days later, streaks of bruises gravitated into the muscles of my thighs and calves, a visible testimonial of the deep tears in my legs. For a week I was unable to wear high heels and I covered the bruises in my legs with dark pantyhose. Two weeks later, I received my black belt at a special ceremony.

I learned a lot from this exhausting weekend. To my surprise, I realized that I could block both my pain and my emotions for long periods of time. For pain control I found myself using two techniques. One was to focus on a certain point, either a part of my body or something in the surrounding environment. This would distract me as I was switching my attention away from the painful event, as well as dissociating my emotional response to pain from my sensory experience of an injurious stimulus.

My second pain-blocking technique was probably mediated through "stress-induced analgesia." At the peak of brutal contact fighting, not only was adrenaline pouring into me, but so were pain-blocking endorphins. This flood of "internal morphines" that humans carry, coupled with attentional switch—you are busy focusing on hitting "fast, hard and first"—obviously made me insensitive to the hits and blows during this crucial period of contact fighting.

I often ponder my professional and personal life. I'm a pain doctor treating other people's pain, but I also know pain first-hand, in both chronic and acute forms. I have spent nearly half of the 20 years of my career in chronic low back pain, and the other half in episodic pain, arising from injuries during my training or my other vigorous physical activities. I did not ask for my back pain, but as my assistant Anna says, I consciously and willingly continue to submit myself to aggressive physical activities, which are frequently accompanied by injuries. So it was also inevitable that I had to devise ways to subdue my pains if I wanted to continue my aggressive lifestyle. No question—pain and I, so often and in so many forms and different types of encounters, are inseparable.

I am fortunate, though, in that I have lived and practised during an explosion of pain science and management.

Our understanding of pain has evolved in a crescendo during the last 200 years, and I don't think we have reached the peak. (Perhaps we never will.) Our probing into what pain means and how to address it systematically started slowly and hesitantly, from the discovery of morphine in the nineteenth century. It has progressed with explosive power and speed during the past 40 years. It seems hard to believe, but before 1960 there were no pain specialists. Major textbooks in medicine and surgery rarely mentioned pain and pain management, and the only pain book (Bonica's *Management of Pain*, published in 1953) was the work of a single man.[1]

In 1960, this one man, Dr. John Bonica, became the chairman of anesthesiology at the University of Washington and from this position he began an international campaign on behalf of pain research and management. Around that time the U.S. National Institute of Health stepped up its general funding for research, and shortly after, in 1965, Melzack and Wall published their gate-control theory, affecting pain research profoundly.

In the 1970s, the pain movement really got off the ground, with the first International Pain Symposium, held in Washington D.C., in 1973. Out of this was born the International Association for the Study of Pain (IASP). Scientific pain journals began appearing, forums where researchers could publish their specialized pain studies, while the milestone of endorphin discovery occurred in 1976. The biological/psychological/sociological approach to pain emerged as an alternative to the strict biomedical approach, and multidisciplinary clinics started sprouting up. One might say that this is when people really began looking beyond pain.

The 1980s saw an explosion in pain research. Standards for training of health care providers and patient care were established, palliative care for cancer patients became a specialty of its own and pain management became a major issue. In the United States, "managed care" and the rationing of health care became hot topics for the media and for politicians, while other countries worried about different forms of cutting costs for their publicly funded programs. In basic science, animal models of pain started making their way through laboratories. Molecular biological approaches, as well as the seeds of understanding the control of pain from the brain and the spinal cord, expanded the knowledge of biological mechanisms of pain.

By the 1990s, the molecular biology of pain continued to thrive, while powerful imaging techniques (fMRI and PET scanning), which could show the thinking and feeling brain in patients who are awake, offered new ways of looking at brain function from a cognitive and psychological point of view. The biopsychosocial model that emerged in the 1980s became widely accepted. The "opium wars" (over the use of opiates) moved from China to North America, and pain, suffering, pain behaviours and disability by this time were hotly debated issues among the experts.

As discussed in Chapter twelve, pain was designated the fifth vital sign in the United States in 1999—a designation that should not be underestimated. In 2000, the U.S. Congress declared the first decade of the twenty-first century to be the "Decade of Pain Awareness and Research."

Where are we going from here? I have no doubt that the neurosciences, including pain science, will continue to develop exponentially. This is not going to be just because of scientific motivation; the pharmaceutical industry has an incentive to develop new drugs for profit. Scientists will continue to target the ways in which injury to tissue is translated into nociception, by looking at channels within the cell membranes and receptors and recording the changes in the nervous system that occur after nerve damage. We will discover new messengers and communication systems between nerve cells or within them, as well as the genes that regulate them.

This is happening already. Recently, the media heralded the discovery of a particular protein, called DREAM (downstream regulatory element antagonistic modulation), that is able to modulate pain.[2] Studies into the circuits that alter the transmission of pain in the brain and the spinal cord will continue, while more sophisticated imaging techniques will shed further light into the mysteries of the mind-body interaction.

For clinical sciences, one of the most important steps will be the development of clinical guidelines for diagnosing and managing chronic painful conditions based on the best evidence available in the literature (similar to the ones developed by CPSO in Ontario). Treatments will have to be judged not only by individuals reporting on their own relief, but by outcomes that can be objectively measured, as those who pay for the care of patients with chronic pain, whether they be insurers, government agencies or individuals, would like to know where their dollars go. While self-reporting is one way to understand how much pain one feels, the success of a given treatment will have to be measured by the activity one can do, how much health care one uses or the capacity the individual has to function in the workplace. Such measurable outcomes then can justify spending money on successful treatments or not spending it on treatments that do not work.

At the same time, we need to improve the way we deal with pain and disability issues, as our understanding moves away from the strict concept of mere bodily injury. Pain and disability must be understood and accepted within their socio-economic context as well. We also need to prevent pain from being generated or from becoming chronic, while at the same time we must treat those who hurt with humane and caring approaches based on the best available knowledge research has taught us. There are many aspects of treatment we should be revisiting in order to reduce the occurrence of chronic pain, for example, how to better avoid unnecessary surgeries, or how to apply aggressive and early management of pain when it occurs.

Hospital and government administrators have a role to play too. If we are to move beyond pain, the health care policy-makers, clinics and institutions will have to provide more funding for treating the psychosocial aspects of pain and disability in multidisciplinary contexts, rather than merely funding procedures like surgery or nerve blocks.

Finally, one of the most important keys to moving beyond pain is education—educating both those who provide care and those of us who suffer from pain. Pain sufferers need to be partners in their own care, aware of what is available and how to use health care resources rationally.

Given the complex nature of chronic pain and the interplay between physical damage, our minds and our interactions with our surroundings, multidisciplinary approaches addressing both the mind and the body will be more successful than isolated pharmacological, psychological, medical or surgical interventions. In the end, it really comes down to people.

Pain management will always need caring and compassionate physicians and health care practitioners, who must keep abreast of scientific developments.

Notes

CHAPTER ONE

[1] Osterweis M, Kleinman A, Mechanic D, editors. Pain and disability: clinical, behavioral and public policy perspectives. Institute of Medicine, Committee on Pain, Disability and Chronic Illness Behavior. Washington D.C.: National Academy Press, 1987.

[2] Mechanic D. The concept of illness behavior. J Chronic Dis 1962;15:189–194.

[3] Osterweis M, Kleinman A, Mechanic D. Pain and disability: clinical, behavioral and public policy perspectives. Institute of Medicine, Committee on Pain, Disability and Chronic Illness Behavior. Washington D.C.: National Academy Press, 1987.

[4] Crook J, Rideout E, Browne G. The prevalence of pain complaints in a general population. Pain 1984;18:299–314.

[5] Bain ST, Spaulding WB. The importance of coding presenting symptoms. Can Med Assoc J 1967;97:953–959.

[6] Crook J, Rideout E, Browne G. The prevalence of pain complaints in a general population. Pain 1984;18:299–314.

[7] Tunks E, Bellissimo A. Chronic pain: the psychotherapeutic spectrum. Praeger Publishers, 1984.

[8] Merskey H, Spear FG. Pain: psychological and psychiatric aspects. London: Balliere, Tindall and Cassell; 1967.

[9] Melzack R, Scott TH. The effects of early experience on the response to pain. J Comp Physiol Psychol 1957;50:155–161.

[10] Tunks E, Bellissimo A. Chronic pain: the psychotherapeutic spectrum. Praeger Publishers, 1984.

[11] Beecher HK. Measurement of subjective responses. New York: Oxford University Press; 1959.

[12] Carlen PL, Wall PD, Nadvorna H, Steinbach T. Phantom limbs and related phenomena in recent traumatic amputations. Neurol 1978;28:211–217.

[13] Pavlov IP. Conditioned reflexes. Oxford: Humphrey Milford; 1927.

[14] Brandt P, Yancey P. Pain: the gift nobody wants. New York: HarperCollins; 1993.

[15] Wynn Parry CB. Pain in avulsion lesions of the brachial plexus. Pain 1980;9: 41–53.

[16] Tunks E, Bellissimo A. Chronic pain: the psychotherapeutic spectrum. Praeger Publishers; 1984.

[17] Lesse S. The multivariant masks of depression. Am J Psychiatry, 1968;124 (Suppl):35–40.

[18] Bates MS. Biocultural dimensions of chronic pain. SUNY series in Medical Anthropology, State University of New York Press; 1996.

[19] Morris DB. Ethnicity and pain. Pain Clinical Updates, Vol. IX, no 4, 2001 Nov.

[20] Mendoza R et al. Psychopharmacol Bull 1991;27:449–461.

[21] Zhou HH et al. Clin Pharmacol Ther 1993; 54:507–513.

[22] Rosmus C et al. Soc Sci Med 2000;51:175–184.

[23] Zborowski M. Cultural components in responses to pain. J Soc Issues, 1952;8: 16–30.

[24] Hardy JD, Wolff HG, Goodell H. Pain sensations and reactions. Baltimore: Williams and Wilkins; 1952.

[25] Sternbach RA, Tursky B. Ethnic differences among housewives in psychophysical and skin potential responses to electric shock. Psychophysiol 1965;1:241–246.

[26] Lambert WE, Libman E, Poser EG. Effect of increased salience of membership group on pain tolerance. J Personality 1960;28:350–357.

[27] Bates MS. Biocultural dimensions of chronic pain. SUNY series in Medical Anthropology, State University of New York Press; 1996.

[28] Coreil J, Marshall PA. Locus of illness control: a cross-cultural study. Human Organizations 1982;41:131–138.

[29] Bates MS. Biocultural dimensions of chronic pain. SUNY series in Medical Anthropology, State University of New York Press; 1996.

[30] Melzack, R, Wall PD, The puzzle of pain. Penguin; 1982.

[31] Morris DB. Ethnicity and pain. Pain Clinical Updates, Vol. IX, no 4, 2001 Nov.

[32] Morrison RS et al. N Engl J Med 2000;342:1023–1026.

[33] De Palma A. For Mexicans, pain relief is both a medical and a political problem. New York Times; 1996 June 19;Sect A:4.

CHAPTER TWO

[1] Merskey H, Bogduk N, editors. Classification of chronic pain syndromes. 2nd ed. Seattle: IASP Press; 1994: p 210.

[2] Pain and disability. Clinical, Behavioral and Public Policy Perspectives. Institute of Medicine, National Academy Press, Washington D.C. 1987.

[3] Melzack R, Wall P. The challenge of pain. Penguin; 1982.

[4] Melzack R, Wall P. The challenge of pain. Penguin; 1982.

[5] Melzack R, Wall P. The challenge of pain. Penguin; 1982.

[6] Mogil JS. The genetic mediation of individual differences in sensitivity to pain and its inhibition. Proc Natl Acad Sci USA 1999;96:7744–7751; Mogil JS. Interactions between sex and genotype in the mediation and modulation of nociception in rodents. In: Fillingim RB, editor. Sex, gender and pain. Progress in pain research and management, Vol. 17. Seattle: IASP Press; 2000: p 25–40; Mogil JS. Individual differences in pain: moving beyond the "universal" rat. APS Bulletin 1999;9:5.

[7] Indo Y, Tsurata Y, Karim MA et al. Mutations in the TPKA/NGF receptor gene in patients with congenital insensitivity to pain with anhidrosis. Nat Genet 1996;13:485–488.

[8] Joutel A, Bousser M-G, Biousse V et al. A gene for familial hemiplegic migraine maps to chromosome 19. Nat Genet 1993;5:40–45.

⁹ Mogil JS. Interactions between sex and genotype in the mediation and modulation of nociception in rodents. In: Fillingim RB, editor. Sex, gender and pain. Progress in pain research and management, Vol. 17. Seattle: IASP Press; 2000: p 25–40.

¹⁰ Devor M, Raber P. Heritability of symptoms in an experimental model of neuropathic pain. Pain 1990;42:51–67.

¹¹ Mailis A, Wade J. Profile of Caucasian women with possible genetic predisposition to reflex sympathetic dystrophy: a pilot study. Clin J Pain 1994;10:210–217.

¹² Kemler MA, van de Vusse AC, van den Berg-Loonen EM et al. HLA-DQ1 associated with reflex sympathetic dystrophy. Neurol 1999;53:1350–1351.

¹³ Mailis A, Wade J. Genetic considerations in CRPS. In: Harden NR, Baron R, Jänig W editors. Complex regional pain syndrome. Progress in pain research and management, Vol. 22. Seattle: IASP Press; 2001: p 227–238.

¹⁴ Price DD. Psychological mechanisms of pain and analgesia. Progress in pain research and management, Vol. 15. Seattle: IASP Press; 1999.

¹⁵ Forth W, Martin E, Peter K. The relief of pain. Hoescht Meducation Update, 1986 Hoechst Aktiengesellschaft.

¹⁶ Melzack R, Wall PD. Pain mechanisms: a new theory. Science 1965;150: 971–979; Melzack R and Wall P. The challenge of pain. Penguin; 1982.

¹⁷ Wall PD. Pain in context: The intellectual roots of pain research and therapy. In: Devor M, Rowbotham MC, Wiesenfeld-Hallin Z editors. Proceedings of the 9th World Congress on Pain. Progress in pain research and management, Vol. 16. Seattle: IASP Press; 2000.

¹⁸ Davis KD, Kwan CL, Crawley AP, Mikulis DJ. Functional MRI study of thalamic and cortical activations. J Neurophysiol 1998;80:1533–1546.

¹⁹ McMurray GA. Experimental study of a case of insensitivity to pain. Arch Neurol Psychiat 1950;64:650–667.

²⁰ Baxter DW, Olszewski J. Congenital insensitivity to pain. Brain 1960;83: 381–393.

²¹ Mailis A. Is diabetic autonomic neuropathy protective against reflex sympathetic dystrophy? Clin J Pain 1995;11:76–84.

CHAPTER THREE

1 Fillingim RB. Sex, gender and pain: a biopsychosocial framework. In: Fillingim RB, editor. Sex, gender and pain. Progress in pain research and management, Vol. 17. Seattle: IASP Press; 2000: p 1–6.

2 Fillingim RB, Maixner W. Gender differences in the responses to noxious stimuli. Pain Forum 1995;4(4):209–221; Unruh AM. Gender variations in clinical pain experience. Pain 1996;65(2–3):123–167; Berkley KJ. Sex differences in pain. Behav Brain Sci 1997;20:371–380.

3 Fillingim RB, Maixner W. Gender differences in the responses to noxious stimuli. Pain Forum 1995;4(4):209–221.

4 LeResche L. Epidemiological perspectives on sex differences in pain. In: Fillingim. RB, editor. Sex, gender and pain. Progress in pain research and management, Vol. 17. Seattle: IASP Press; 2000: p 233–249.

5 Engel G. A unified concept of health and disease. Perspect Biol Med 1960;3:459–485.

6 Robinson ME, Riley JL III, Myers C. Psychosocial contributions to sex related differences in pain responses. In: Fillingim RB, editor. Sex, gender and pain. Progress in pain research and management, Vol. 17. Seattle: IASP Press; 2000: p 41–68.

7 Moir A, Jessel D. Brain sex. Mandarin; 1991.

8 Garai JE, Scheinfeld A. Sex differences in mental and behavioral traits. Genetic Psychology Monographs, 1968;77:169–299.

9 Lloyd B, Archer J. Sex and gender, London: Penguin; 1982.

10 Lloyd B, Archer J. Sex and gender, London: Penguin; 1982.

11 Lloyd B, Archer J. Sex and gender, London: Penguin; 1982.

12 Lloyd B, Archer J. Sex and gender, London: Penguin; 1982.

13 Aloisi AM. Sensory effects of gonadal hormones. In: Fillingim RB, editor. Sex, gender and pain. Progress in pain research and management, Vol. 17. Seattle: IASP Press; 2000: p 7–24.

14 Rizzolatti G, Buchtel HA. Hemispheric superiority in reaction time to faces: a sex difference. Cortex 1977;13:300–305.

[15] Robinson E, Short RV. Changes in breast sensitivity at puberty, during the menstrual cycle and at parturition. BMJ 1977;7:1188–1191.

[16] Aloisi AM. Sensory effects of gonadal hormones. In: Fillingim RB, editor. Sex, gender and pain. Progress in pain research and management, Vol. 17. Seattle: IASP Press; 2000: p 7–24.

[17] Moir A, Jessel D. Brain sex. Mandarin; 1991.

[18] Moir A, Jessel D. Brain sex. Mandarin; 1991.

[19] Witleson SF. Sex differences in the neurology of cognition: social, educational and clinical implications. In: Sulleror E, editor. Le fait feminin Fayard, France 1978:287–303.

[20] Aloisi AM. Sensory effects of gonadal hormones. In: Fillingim RB, editor. Sex, gender and pain. Progress in pain research and management, Vol. 17. Seattle: IASP Press; 2000: p 7–24.

[21] Walker JS, Carmody JJ. Experimental pain in healthy human subjects: gender differences in nociception and in response to ibuprofen. Anesth Analg 1998;86:1257–1262.

[22] Miaskowski C, Gear RW, Levine JD. Sex-related differences in analgesic responses. In: Fillingim RB, editor. Sex, gender and pain. Progress in pain research and management, Vol. 17. Seattle: IASP Press; 2000: p 209–230.

[23] Gintzler AR, Liu N-J. Ovarian sex steroids activate antinociceptive systems and reveal gender-specific mechanisms. In: Fillingim RB, editor. Sex, gender and pain. Progress in pain research and management, Vol. 17. Seattle: IASP Press; 2000: p 89–108.

[24] Komisaruk BR, Whipple B. How does vaginal stimulation produce pain, pleasure and analgesia? In: Fillingim RB, editor. Sex, gender and pain. Progress in pain research and management, Vol. 17. Seattle: IASP Press; 2000: p 109–134.

[25] LeResche L. Gender, cultural and environmental aspects of pain. In: Loeser JD, Butler SH, Chapman CR, Turk DC, editors. Bonica's management of pain. 3rd ed. Lippincott Williams & Wilkins; 2001: p 191–195.

[26] Robinson ME, Riley JL III, Myers C. Psychosocial contributions to sex-related differences in pain responses. In: Fillingim RB, editor. Sex, gender and pain. Progress in pain research and management, Vol. 17. Seattle: IASP Press; 2000: p 41–68.

[27] Klonoff EA, Landrine H. Culture and gender diversity beliefs about the causes of six illnesses. J Behav Med 1994;17(4):407–418.

[28] Levine FM, De Simone LL. The effects of experimenter gender on pain report in male and female subjects. Pain 1991;44:69–72; Feine JS, Bushnell MC, Miron D, Duncan GH. Sex differences in the perception of noxious heat stimuli. Pain 1991;44:255–262.

[29] Lash SJ, Eisler RM, Schulman RS. Cardiovascular reactivity to stress in men: effects of masculine gender role stress appraisal and masculine performance challenge. Behav Modif 1990;14(1):3–20.

[30] Robinson ME, Riley JL III, Myers C. Psychosocial contributions to sex-related differences in pain responses. In: Fillingim RB, editor. Sex, gender and pain. Progress in pain research and management, Vol. 17. Seattle: IASP Press; 2000: p 41–68.

[31] Turk DC, Rudy TE. Assessment of cognitive factors in chronic pain: a worthwhile enterprise? J Consult Clin Psychol 1986;54(6):760–768.

[32] Nolen-Hoeksema S. Sex differences in depression. Stanford: Stanford University Press; 1990.

[33] Bolton JE. Psychological distress and disability in back pain patients: evidence of sex differences. J Psychosom Res 1994;38(8):849–858.

[34] Lacroix R, Barbaree HE. The impact of recurrent headaches on behavior lifestyle and health. Behav Res Ther 1990;28(3):235–242; Gilbar O, Bazak Y, Harel Y. Gender, primary headache, and psychological distress. Headache 1998;38(1):31–34.

CHAPTER FOUR

[1] Soo YS, Singh J. Some radiological observations on the practice of insertion of "charm needles." Med J Malaysia 1972;27:40–42.

[2] Hopkins E. Encyclopedia of religion and ethics. New York: Scribners; 1913;6: p 30–31.

[3] Frazer J. The golden bough: A study of magic and religion, 3rd ed. London: Macmillan & Co: vol.V, Bk 1, Ch 5, p 115, and vol.V, Bk 1, Ch 6, p 169, 1911–1915.

[4] Mysteries of the unknown. Mind over body. Alexandria, VA: Time-Life Books; 1988: p 102–120.

[5] Price H. Fire walking experiments: report on Kuda Bux's demonstration. Br Med J 1935;2:586.

[6] Darling CR. Fire-walking (correspondence), Nature, 1935 Sept 28.

[7] Thomas ES. Fire-walking. Nature, 1936 Feb 8; 213–215.

[8] Fonseca C. Fire-walking: a scientific investigation. Ceylon Med J 1971 June; 104–109.

[9] Wijeywardene G. Fire-walking and the scepticism of Varro. Caberra Anthropology, 1979;2:114–133.

[10] Obeyesekere G. The fire-walkers of Kataragama: the rise of Bahkti religiosity in Buddhist Sri Lanka. J Asian Stud 1987;37:463–466.

[11] Browne DRG. Ritual and pain. In: Man RD editor. The history of the management of pain. Park Ridge, NJ: Parthenon Publishing Group; 1988: p 31–49.

[12] Larbig W, Lutzenberger W, Elbert T, Rochstroh B, Birbaumer N. EEG and slow cortical potentials related to laboratory pain and EEG correlates of pain during firewalking in Greece. Pain 1981; Suppl. 1, 557; Larbig W, Haag G, Birbaumer N. Pain regulation and psychosomatics: Preliminary experiments and field studies in fire-walkers. In: Zander W, editor. Experimentelle Forschungs-ergebnisse in der psychosomatischen Medizin. Gottingen: Vandenhoeck and Ruprecht; 1981: p 59–68; Larbig W. Schmerz. Grundlagen – Forschung – Therapie. Stuttgart, Berlin, Cologne and Mainz: Verlag W. Kohlhammer; 1982; p 190–199, 269.

[13] Inglis B. Through the heat barrier. Guardian, 1985 June 5; Thynne J. Bromiley quoted in Hot foot shuffle. Sunday Times, 1985 June 16;36.

[14] Thynne J. Bromiley quoted in Hot foot shuffle. Sunday Times, 1985 June 16;36.

[15] Browne DRG. Ritual and pain. In: Man RD, editor. The history of the management of pain. Park Ridge, NJ: Parthenon Publishing Group; 1988: p 31–49.

[16] Larbig W, Haag G, Birbaumer N. Pain regulation and psychosomatics: preliminary experiments and field studies in fire-walkers. In: Zander W, editor. Experimentelle Forschungs-ergebnisse in der psychosomatischen Medizin, Gottingen: Vandenhoeck and Ruprecht; 1981: p 59–68; Larbig W. Schmerz. Grundlagen – Forschung – Therapie. Stuttgart, Berlin, Cologne and Mainz: Verlag W. Kohlhammer; 1982: p 190–199, 269.

[17] Browne DRG. Ritual and pain. In: Man RD, editor. The history of the management of pain. Park Ridge, NJ: Parthenon Publishing Group; 1988: p 31–49.

[18] Obeyesekere G. Medusa's hair London: University of Chicago Press; 1981: p 142–149.

[19] Browne DRG. Ritual and pain. In: Man RD, editor. The history of the management of pain, Park Ridge, NJ: Parthenon Publishing Group; 1988: p 31–49.

[20] Browne DRG. Ritual and pain. In: Man RD, editor. The history of the management of pain. Park Ridge, NJ: Parthenon Publishing Group; 1988: p 31–49.

[21] Fonseca C. The mystery of the hanging Kavadi. The Nation 1973 Mar 16.

[22] Fraioli F, Moretti C, Paolucci D, Alicicco F, Crescenzi F, Fortunio G. Physical exercise stimulates marked concomitant release of β-endorphin and adrenocorticotropic hormone (ACTH) in peripheral blood in man. Experientia 1980;36:987–989.

[23] Janal MN, Cort EWD, Clark WC, Glusman M. Pain sensitivity and plasma endocrine levels in man following long-distance running: effects of naloxone. Pain 1984;19:13–25.

[24] Crapanzano V. The Hamadsha: a study in Moroccan ethno psychiatry. London: University of California Press; 1973, p 185–211, 231–235.

[25] Anand BK, Chhina GS, Singh B. Some aspects of electroencephalographic studies in yogis. Electroenceph Clin Neurophysiol 1961;13:452–456.

[26] Wall PD. Foreword to the 1983 Edition. Hilgard ER, Hilgard JR. Hypnosis in the relief of pain. William Kaufmann; 1983.

[27] Hadfield A. The influence of hypnotic suggestions on inflammatory conditions. Lancet 1917;2:678–679.

[28] Moody RL. Bodily changes during abreaction. Lancet 1946:934-935 and 1948:964.

[29] Mysteries of the unknown. Mind over body. Alexandria, VA: Time-Life Books; 1988: p 102–120.

[30] Mysteries of the unknown. Mind over body. Alexandria, VA: Time-Life Books; 1988: p 102–120.

[31] Barber J. Hypnosis and suggestion in the treatment of pain. New York: Norton; 1996.

[32] Kiernan BD, Dane JR, Phillips LH et al. Hypnotic analgesia reduces R-III nociceptive reflex; further evidence concerning the multifactorial nature of hypnotic analgesia. Pain 1995;60:39–47.

[33] Price DD. Psychological mechanisms of pain and analgesia. In: Progress in pain research and management, Vol. 15. Seattle: IASP Press; 1999.

[34] Brody H. Placebo effect: an examination of Grünbaum's definition. In: White L, Tursky B, Schwartz GE, editors. Placebo: theory, research and mechanisms. New York: Guilford Press; 1985: p 37–58.

[35] Beecher HK. The powerful placebo. JAMA 1955;159:1602–1606.

[36] Roberts AH, Kewman DG, Mercier L et al. The power of non-specific effects in healing: implications for psychosocial and biological treatments. Clin Psychol Rev 1993;13:375–391.

[37] Cobb LA, Thomas GI, Dillard DH et al. An evaluation of internal-mammary-artery-ligation by a double blind technic. N Engl J Med 1959;260: 1115–1118.

[38] Schweiger A, Parducci A. Nocebo: the psychologic induction of pain. Pavlov J Biol Sci 1981;16:140–143.

[39] Benedetti F, Pollo A. The pharmacology of placebos. Intern J Pain Med Pall Care 2001(1);2:42–48.

CHAPTER FIVE

[1] Frank J, Sinclair S, Hogg-Johnson S, Shannon H, Bombardier C, Beaton D et al. Preventing disability from work-related low-back pain: new evidence gives new hope—if we can just get all the players onside. CMAJ 1998;158(12):1625–1631.

CHAPTER SIX

[1] Evans DP. Backache: its evolution and conservative treatment. Baltimore: University Park Press; 1982.

[2] Bigos SJ and Müller G. Primary care approach to acute and chronic back problems: definitions and care. In: Loeser DJ, Butler SH, Chapman CR, Turk DC, editors. Bonica's management of pain. 3rd ed. Lippincott Williams & Wilkins; 2001: p 1509–1528.

[3] Bigos SJ and Müller G. Primary care approach to acute and chronic back problems: definitions and care. In: Loeser DJ, Butler SH, Chapman CR, Turk DC, editors. Bonica's management of pain. 3rd ed. Lippincott Williams & Wilkins; 2001: p 1509–1528.

[4] Waddell G. Social interactions. In: Waddell G, editor. The back pain revolution. New York: Churchill Livingstone; 1998: p 203–223.

[5] Wilkinson HA. The failed back syndrome: etiology and therapy. Philadelphia: Harper & Row; 1983; Finneson BE, Cooper VR. A lumbar disc surgery predictive score card. Spine 1979;4:141–144.

[6] Finneson BE, Cooper VR. A lumbar disc surgery predictive score card. Spine 1979;4:141–144.

[7] Long DM, Filtzer DL, BenDebba M et al. Clinical features of failed back syndrome. J Neurosurg 1988;69:61–71.

[8] Oaklander AL, North R. Failed back surgery syndrome. In: Loeser DJ, Butler SH, Chapman CR, Turk DC, editors. Bonica's management of pain. 3rd ed. Lippincott Williams & Wilkins; 2001: p 1540–1549.

[9] Oaklander AL, North R. Failed back surgery syndrome. In: Loeser DJ, Butler SH, Chapman CR, Turk DC, editors. Bonica's management of pain. 3rd ed. Lippincott Williams & Wilkins; 2001: p 1540–1549.

[10] Canadian Consortium on Pain Mechanisms, Diagnosis and Management, First Annual Report 1999–2000.

[11] College of Physicians and Surgeons of Ontario (CPSO). Evidence-based recommendations for the medical management of chronic non-malignant pain, 2000.

[12] Greenhalgh S. Under the medical gaze. University of California Press; 2001.

[13] Smythe HA, Moldofsky H. Two contributions to understanding of the "fibrositis syndrome." Bull Rheum Dis 1977;28:928–931.

[14] Wolfe F, Smythe HA, Yunus MB et al. The American College of Rheumatology 1990 Criteria for the Classification of Fibromyalgia. Report of the Multicentre Criteria Committee. Arthritis Rheum 1990;33:160–172.

[15] Wolfe F, Ross K, Anderson J, Hebert L. The prevalence and characteristics of fibromyalgia in the general population. Arthr Rheum 1995;38(1):19–28.

[16] Croft P, Schollum J, Silman A. Population study of tender point counts and pain as evidence of fibromyalgia. BMJ 1994;309:696–699.

[17] Tunks E. Nonspecificity of chronic soft tissue pain syndromes. Pain Res Manage 1997; 2(3):176–180.

[18] Smythe HA, Gladman A, Mader R, Peloso P, Abu-Shakra M. Strategies for accessing pain and pain exaggeration: controlled studies. J Rheumatol 1997;24:1622–1629.

[19] Cameron RS. The cost of long term disability due to fibromyalgia, chronic fatigue syndrome and repetitive strain injury: the private insurance perspective. J Musculoskel Pain 1995;3:169–172.

[20] Tunks E. Nonspecificity of chronic soft tissue pain syndromes. Pain Res Manage 1997; 2(3):176–180.

[21] Gracely RH, Petzke F, Wolf JM, Clauw DJ. Functional magnetic resonance imaging evidence of augmented pain processing in fibromyalgia. Arthritis & Rheumatism 2002;46:1333–1343.

[22] Poyhia R, Da Costa D, Fitzcharles MA. Previous pain experience in women with fibromyalgia and inflammatory arthritis and non-painful controls. Rheumatol 2001;28:1888–1891; Katon W, Sullivan M, Walker E. Medical symptoms without identified pathology: relationship to psychiatric disorders, childhood and adult trauma, and personality traits. Ann Intern Med 2001;11:917–925.

[23] Mailis A, Papagapiou M, Umana M, Cohodarevic T, Nowak J, Nicholson K. Unexplainable non-dermatomal somatosensory deficits in patients with chronic non-malignant pain in the context of litigation/compensation: a role for involvement of central factors? J Rheumatol 2001;28:1385–1393; Mailis-Gagnon A, Giannoylis I, Downar J, Kwan CL, Mikulis DJ, Crawley AP, Nicholson K, Davis KD. Altered central somatosensory processing in chronic pain patients with "hysterical anesthesia." Neurology 2003;60:1501–1507.

CHAPTER SEVEN

[1] Mailis A, Amani N, Umana M, Basur R, Roe S. Effects of intravenous sodium amytal on cutaneous sensory abnormalities, spontaneous pain and algometric pain pressure thresholds in neuropathic pain patients: a placebo-controlled study. Pain 1997;70:69–81.

[2] Wesselman U. Management of chronic pelvic pain. In: Aronoff GM, editor. Evaluation and treatment of chronic pain. 3rd ed. Williams & Wilkins; 1998: p 269–279.

3 Wesselman U. Management of chronic pelvic pain. In: Aronoff GM, editor. Evaluation and treatment of chronic pain. 3rd ed. Williams & Wilkins; 1998: p 269–279.

4 Wesselman U. Management of chronic pelvic pain. In: Aronoff GM, editor. Evaluation and treatment of chronic pain. 3rd ed. Williams & Wilkins; 1998: p 269–279.

5 Cannon RO III. Cardiac pain. In: Gebhart GF, editor. Visceral pain. Progress in pain research and management, Vol 5. Seattle: IASP Press; 1995: p 373–389.

6 Rao SSC. Esophageal (noncardiac) chest pain: visceral hyperalgesia, motor disorder, or reflux disease? In: Gebhart GF, editor. Visceral pain. Progress in pain research and management, Vol 5. Seattle: IASP Press; 1995: p 351–371.

7 Cannon RO III. Cardiac pain. In: Gebhart GF, editor. Visceral pain. Progress in pain research and management, Vol 5. Seattle: IASP Press; 1995: p 373–389.

8 Cannon RO III. Cardiac pain. In: Gebhart GF, editor. Visceral pain. Progress in pain research and management, Vol 5. Seattle: IASP Press; 1995: p 373–389.

9 Mailis A, Bennett GJ. Painful neurological disorders: clinical aspects. In: Aronoff GM, editor. Evaluation and treatment of chronic pain. 3rd ed. Williams & Wilkins; 1998: p 93–113.

10 Mailis A, Bennett GJ. Painful neurological disorders: clinical aspects. In: Aronoff GM, editor. Evaluation and treatment of chronic pain. 3rd ed. Williams & Wilkins; 1998: p 93–113.

11 Mailis A, Bennett GJ. Painful neurological disorders: clinical aspects. In: Aronoff GM, editor. Evaluation and treatment of chronic pain. 3rd ed. Williams & Wilkins; 1998: p 93–113.

12 Mailis A, Bennett GJ. Painful neurological disorders: clinical aspects. In: Aronoff GM, editor. Evaluation and treatment of chronic pain. 3rd ed. Williams & Wilkins; 1998: p 93–113.

13 Chan PSL, Clark AJ. Postherpetic neuralgia: review of treatment modalities. Pain Res Manage 2000;5(1):69–74.

14 Chan PSL, Clark AJ. Postherpetic neuralgia: review of treatment modalities. Pain Res Manage 2000;5(1):69–74.

15 Mailis A, Chan J, Basinski A, Feindel C, Vanderlinden G et al. Chest wall pain after aortocoronary bypass surgery using internal mammary artery graft: a new pain syndrome? Heart & Lung 1989;18:553–558.

[16] Mailis A, Umana M, Feindel C. Anterior intercostal nerve damage after CABG-ITA surgery. Ann Thor Surg 2000;69:1455–1458.

[17] Furlan AD, Sandoval JA, Mailis-Gagnon A, Taylor R. Spinal cord stimulators for chronic pain: a systematic review of randomized controlled trials. Cochrane collaboration. Submitted.

CHAPTER EIGHT

[1] Fanciullo GJ, Cobb JL. The use of opioids for chronic non-cancer pain. Intern J Pain Med Pall Care, 2001;1(2):49–55.

[2] Portenoy RK, Foley KM. Chronic use of opioid analgesics in non-malignant pain. Report of 38 cases. Pain 1986;25:171–186.

[3] Harden NR. Chronic opioid therapy: another reappraisal. APS Bulletin 2002;12:1.

[4] Harden NR. Chronic opioid therapy: another reappraisal. APS Bulletin 2002;12:1.

[5] Harden NR. Chronic opioid therapy: another reappraisal. APS Bulletin 2002;12:1.

[6] Rinaldi RC, Steindler EM, Wilford BB, Goodwin D. Clarification and standardization of substance terminology. JAMA 1988;259:555–557.

[7] Zenz M, Strumpf M, Tryba M. Long-term oral opioid therapy in patients with chronic non-malignant pain. J Pain Symptom Manag 1992;7:69–77.

[8] Gevirtz C. The patient undergoing ultrarapid opiate detoxification. Anesthesiol News 2000 June;62:67.

[9] Fishbain DA, Rosomoff HL, Rosomoff RS. Drug abuse, dependence and addiction in chronic pain patients. Clin J Pain 1992;8:77–85.

[10] Fanciullo GJ, Cobb JL. The use of opioids for chronic non-cancer pain. Intern J Pain Med Pall Care 2001;1(2):49–55.

[11] Perry S, Hedrich G. Management of pain during debridement: a survey of US burn units. Pain 1985;13:267–280.

[12] Robins LN, Davis DH, Nurco DN. How permanent was Vietnam addiction? Am J Public Health 1974;64:38–43.

[13] CPSO Evidence-based recommendations for the medical management of chronic non-malignant pain; 2000.

[14] CPSO Evidence-based recommendations for the medical management of chronic non-malignant pain; 2000.

[15] CPSO Evidence-based recommendations for the medical management of chronic non-malignant pain; 2000.

[16] Mogil JS. Interactions between sex and genotype in the mediation and modulation of nociception in rodents. In: Fillingim RB, editor. Sex, gender and pain. Progress in pain research and management, Vol. 17. Seattle: IASP Press; 2000: p 25–40.

[17] Harden NR. Chronic opioid therapy: another reappraisal. APS Bulletin 2002;12:1.

[18] Harden NR. Chronic opioid therapy: another reappraisal. APS Bulletin 2002;12:1.

[19] Harden NR. Chronic opioid therapy: another reappraisal. APS Bulletin 2002;12:1.

[20] Bradley CM, Nicholson AN. Effects of μ-opioid receptor agonist (codeine phosphate) on the visuo-motor coordination and dynamic visual acuity in man. Br J Clin Pharmacol, 1986;22:507; Chapman S. The effects of opioids on driving ability of patients with chronic pain. APS Bulletin 2001;11(1):1, 5, 9; Joranson DE, Gilson AM. State intractable pain policy: current status. APS Bull 1997;7(2):7–9; Payne R. Assessments of analgesic-induced performance deficits. APS Bulletin 1991;1(2):6–9.

[21] Mechoulam R. The cannabinoids: an overview. Therapeutic implications in vomiting and nausea after cancer chemotherapy, in appetite promotion, in multiple sclerosis and neuroptrotection. Pain Res Manage 2001;6(2):67–73.

[22] Kalant H. Medicinal use of cannabis: history and current status. Pain Res Manage 2001;6(2):80–91.

[23] Walker JM, Strangman NM, Huang SM. Cannabinoids and pain. Pain Res Manage 2001;6(2):74–79.

[24] Joy JE, Watson SJ, Benson JA, Jr, editors. Marijuana and medicine: assessing the science base. Washington D.C.: National Academy Press; 1999.

[25] Walker JM, Strangman NM, Huang SM. Cannabinoids and pain. Pain Res Manage 2001;6(2):74–79.

[26] Kalant H. Medicinal use of cannabis: history and current status. Pain Res Manage 2001;6(2):80–91.

CHAPTER NINE

[1] Asher R. Munchausen's syndrome. Lancet 1951;1:339–341.

[2] Meadow R. Suffocation: recurrent apnea and sudden infant death. J Pediatr 1990;117:351–358.

[3] McDonald M. SEPTA does its math homework. Philadelphia Daily News 1988 Sept 28.

[4] Loundsberry E. Doctor 73, lauded as charitable, caring, gets jail for mail fraud. Philadelphia Inquirer 1998 Aug 31.

[5] Malleson A. Whiplash and other useful illnesses. Montreal: McGill-Queen's University Press; 2002: p. 267.

[6] Malleson A. Whiplash and other useful illnesses. Montreal: McGill-Queen's University Press; 2002: p. 268.

[7] "Ghost riders," Eye To Eye with Connie Chung, Produced by J. Martelli, Aug 18, 1992.

[8] Malleson A. Whiplash and other useful illnesses. Montreal: McGill-Queen's University Press; 2002: p. 268.

[9] Gollom M. Five doctors, paralegal charged in insurance scam. National Post 2000 June 7; A24.

[10] Baer N. Fraud worries insurance companies but should concern physicians too, industry says. CMAJ 1997;156:251–253.

[11] Winchell RM, Stanley M. Self-injurious behaviour: a review of the behaviour and biology of self-mutilation. Am J Psychiat 1991;148:306–317.

[12] Winchell RM, Stanley M. Self-injurious behaviour: a review of the behaviour and biology of self-mutilation. Am J Psychiat 1991;148:306–317.

[13] Freeman AG. Trigeminal neuralgia: complications of its surgical treatment. Br Med J 1967;1:631–632.

[14] Mailis A. Compulsive targeted self-injurious behaviour in humans with neuropathic pain: a counterpart of animal autotomy? Four case reports and literature review. Pain 1996;64:569–578.

CHAPTER TEN

[1] Mailis A. Compulsive targeted self-injurious behaviour in humans with neuropathic pain: a counterpart of animal autotomy? Four case reports and literature review. Pain 1996;64:569–578; Mailis A, Plapler P, Ashby P, Shoichet R, Roe S. Effect of intravenous sodium amytal on cutaneous limb temperatures and sympathetic skin responses in normal subjects and pain patients with and without Complex Regional Pain Syndromes (Type I and II). Pain 1997;70:59–68; Mailis A, Amani N, Umana M, Basur R, Roe S. Effects of intravenous sodium amytal on cutaneous sensory abnormalities, spontaneous pain and algometric pain pressure thresholds in neuropathic pain patients: a placebo-controlled study. Pain 1997;70:69–81.

[2] Fishbain DA, Goldberg M, Steele Rosomoff R et al. Chronic pain patients and the nonorganic physical signs of nondermatomal sensory abnormalities. Psychosomatics 1991;32:294–303.

[3] Kaziyama HHS, Texeira MJ, Lin TY et al. Fibromyalgia and hemisensitive syndromes (abstract). IASP 9th World Congress on Pain, Vienna, Austria 1999: p 550.

[4] Mailis A, Papagapiou M, Umana M, Cohodarevic T, Nowak J, Nicholson K. Unexplainable non-dermatomal somatosensory deficits in patients with chronic non-malignant pain in the context of litigation/compensation: a role for involvement of central factors? J Rheumatol 2001;28:1385–1393.

[5] Cohodarevic T, Mailis A, Montanera W. Syringomyelia: pain, somatosensory abnormalities and neuroimaging. J Pain 2000;1(1):54–66.

[6] Mailis-Gagnon A, Giannoylis I, Downar J, Kwan CL, Mikulis DJ, Crawley AP, Nicholson K, Davis KD. Altered central somatosensory processing in chronic pain patients with "hysterical anesthesia." Neurology 2003;60:1501–1507.

[7] Sacks O. A leg to stand on. Touchstone; 1998.

CHAPTER ELEVEN

[1] Fishbain, D, Bruns, Trape M. Chronic pain patients' risk for violent behavior: evaluation and management in the pain facility setting. American Pain Society 19th Annual Meeting, 2000: p 71.

[2] Mailis A; Wade JA. Clinical profiles of female patients with genetic predisposition to RSD: a pilot study. Clin J Pain 1994;10:210–217.

CHAPTER TWELVE

[1] Catchlove RFH, Hoirsch AM. Survey of Canadian pain centres: a preliminary report. Pain Clinic 1988;2:231–237.

[2] Cleland LG. RSI: a model of social iatrogenesis. Medical Journal of Australia 1987;147:236–239; Bell DS. Repetition strain injury: an iatrogenic epidemic of simulated injury. Medical Journal of Australia 1989;151:280–284.

[3] Raffle PAB. Automation and repetitive work: their effect on health. Lancet 1963;1:733–737.

[4] Bell DS. Repetition strain injury: an iatrogenic epidemic of simulated injury. Medical Journal of Australia 1989;151:280–284; Littlejohn GO. Key issues in repetitive strain injury. Journal of Musculoskeletal Pain 1995;3:25–33.

[5] Bell DS. Repetition strain injury: an iatrogenic epidemic of simulated injury. Medical Journal of Australia 1989;151:280–284.

[6] Bigos SJ, Battié MC. The impact of spinal dosorders in industry. In: Frymoyer JW et al, editors. The adult spine: principles and practice. New York: Raven Press; 1991: p 147–154 (Ch.9); Frank JW et al. Occupational back pain: an unhelpful polemic. Scand J Wor Environ Health 1995;21:3–14.

[7] Malleson A. Whiplash and other useful illnesses. Montreal: McGill-Queen's University Press; 2002: p 93–101.

[8] Agency for Health Care Policy and Research. Clinical practice guideline. Number 14: acute low back problems in adults. Rockville, MD: Department of Health and Human Services; 1992.

[9] Decter M. Four strong winds. Toronto: Stoddart; 2000.

[10] Buchbinder R, Jolley D, Wyatt M. 2001 Volvo Award winner in clinical studies: Effects of a media campaign on back pain beliefs and its potential influence on management of low back pain in general practice. Spine 2001;16:2535–2542.

[11] Cassidy DJ, Carroll LJ et al. Effect of eliminating compensation for pain and suffering on the outcome of insurance claims for whiplash injury. N Engl J Med 2000;342:1179–1186.

[12] Van Voris B. No gain, no pain? National Law Journal 2000 May 22:1.

[13] Furlan A, Mailis A, Papagapiou M. Are we paying a high price for surgical sympathectomy? A systematic literature review of late complications. J Pain 2000;1(4):245–257.

EPILOGUE

[1] Loeser, JD. The future: will pain be abolished or just pain management specialists? Pain Clinical Updates, Vol. VIII. IASP; 2000 Dec 6.

[2] Cheng MHY et al. DREAM is a critical transcriptional repressor for pain modulation. Cell 2002;108:31–43.

Case Studies

* All names used for case studies are pseudonyms, except for Alex
  (son of Angela Mailis-Gagnon) and Norm (her husband)

Name Index

Subject Index